All dentists want their patient to like them and come again. All patients want to like their dentist, but hope they never have to come again. Talk about different agendas! Dentists are trained to help patients prevent dental disease wherever possible and treat dental conditions as early as possible, yet their practices are often based on treating long-standing disease and conditions or repairing breakdown that has been left unattended for some time. These last two approaches to dental care are the most costly for the patient, yet provide the bulk of income for almost every dental practice. In a perfect world, patients assume responsibility for themselves. They don't remove bottle caps or drag 18-wheelers with their teeth. They eat healthy foods and avoid Sugar Daddies, Mountain Dew, and foods that contribute directly to tooth decay. They regularly clean their teeth. They seek the advice and care of a dentist to avoid problems and address conditions before they become costly and catastrophic. They demand preventative care such as cleanings, x-rays, sealants, and rinses. But it isn't a perfect world. Too often, patients avoid or delay care, resulting in more serious conditions with the most costly and extreme solutions. On top of that, many people who have not sought care are embarrassed to have a dentist see the dire straits in which they find themselves. Pain, shame, fear, financial limitations, embarrassment—all powerful factors which must be recognized, addressed, and handled gently by the dentist who is asked to help a patient in distress. Very special circumstances require a very special dentist—one who is highly competent as a clinician and also highly competent as a human being. This combination is rare, but Dr. Randy Mitchmore is the finest example on both fronts. In this book, you will read story after story of ordinary people whose lives he has touched in a meaningful way. And, you will learn of his struggles and what he did to overcome the challenges of life. These experiences have made him the human being and, therefore, the dentist, he is today. As a father, partner, public servant, professional clinician, and humanitarian, Dr. Mitchmore is a role model for his peers. He is admired by many and respected by all. I'm sure you will enjoy reading about him and his journey. May it inspire you in your own life.

—SANDY ROTH, Owner of ProSynergy, consultant to the dental profession, especially in communication and organization, former Philadelphia police officer transformed to a Master Teacher, www.prosynergy.com

Dr. Mitchmore has done a wonderful job of showing his passion for the profession he loves. It is this passion that drives him to be in the top 3 percent of dentists. He has exposed several truths about dentistry. This is a must read for anyone who values their dental health.

—BILL BLATCHFORD, DDS, coach, speaker, and author

Dr. Randy Mitchmore's passion and compassion are omnipresent throughout this book. He generously shares information about dentistry that every consumer should know.

More importantly, he weaves the journey of patients' and his own individual story to bring authenticity to a journey of discovery and how to reach the dream of greater confidence, better performance, and reaching your own personal dreams. I highly recommend this book to anyone who seeks learn about the finest that dentistry can provide.

—HUGH FLAX, DDS, AAACD, FICOI, President 2010-2011, American Academy of Cosmetic Dentistry (www.AACD.com), Atlanta, GA

Dr. Randy Mitchmore's new book, The Gift of a Life Smile, *is outstanding. It shows patients how to select dentists who provide outstanding dentistry in a caring environment. In addition, the book gives dentists the information needed to build relationship-driven practices that provide this exceptional care and are professionally fulfilling to lead.*

All of this is wrapped around Randy's personal and extremely unique story. I'm thrilled to be part of Randy's journey as one of his teachers and colleagues. You must read The Gift of a Life Smile. *It will be a glorious gift for you to enhance your health, well-being and happiness or your dental practice.*

—DR. ARUN K. GARG, Founder and CEO of Implant Seminars, President of the International Dental Implant Association

They say when you look deeply into a persons face you can see their life flash before you. Like one of those sci-fi movies where you watch a movie in the minds eye in reverse as you hear and see how a person becomes who they are.

Each story, just like your life, like your smile, is unique. Like a painting, one-of-a-kind, something you can call all your own.

In this book Dr. Randy Mitchmore provides this look back into the lives of his patients and of himself and you get to read everything that goes into a Life Smile. Dr. Mitchmore, like a commissioned artist takes the beautiful person that lives within you and creates the most extraordinary beauty and spirit shown brightly by your new smile.

When you read the culmination of his life's work (don't worry, he's far from finished). Take time to relate to your own personal journey, the stages and phases of your own personal development, the triumphs and tragedies of your life's expedition that has led you to where you are today.

You will soon feel, and I use that word very deliberately, the impact that Dr. Mitchmore has had on his patient's lives and the impact Dr. Mitchmore's patients have had on his.

As the worlds foremost authority on Entrepreneurship, Business Development and Marketing Strategist I can attest to the fact that no person can get to where they want to go or become who they wish to be on their own. My clients need me to guide and help to create the business they dream of having and vice versa, I need them, without clients to serve I am purposeless.

And that my friends, is exactly the case with Dr. Mitchmore. You are about to discover a Man on a mission to change your life. His purpose goes so far beyond the external beauty of the smile you will see in the mirror, more than this is how alive you will feel, how empowered you will be, and how vibrantly your spirit and confidence with shine through.

When you choose whom you go to for advice, leadership, a talent or expertise such as with Dentistry you are looking for more than just a Doctor, you want a friend. You want to find someone who makes you feel comfortable, that you can confide in, that has experienced their own life struggles and overcome.

Dr. Mitchmore likes to say "go with your gut" and trust yourself. You will know because you will feel it, in your hands as you read this book, and in your soul when you begin your relationship with Dr. Mitchmore and his amazing team.

He calls his proprietary approach and the result of what you will receive a "Life Smile" and that is the most fitting phrase he could have ever come up with because you are making a Life decision, one that you will never forget and always remember what it was like before and after you made the commitment to live the life you were meant to live.

They say you can judge a person by the integrity they have and the company they keep. Inside this book Dr. Mitchmore brings you a transparent look at his journey through finding himself and helping his patients do the same.

You are amongst good company when you walk into Dr. Mitchmore's office. I assure you there's no one better in all the world to be your guide on this journey of creating Your Life Smile than Dr. Randy Mitchmore.

—SCOTT MANNING, MBA - **Founder of Million Dollar Methods and Coach to the Coaches for Entrepreneurs world wide.**

The GIFT of a
LIFE SMILE

The GIFT of a LIFE SMILE

Your Guide *to* Uncovering
Your White Smile *and* Hidden Happiness

DR. RANDY MITCHMORE, DDS, MAGD

Advantage®

Published by Advantage, Charleston, South Carolina.
Member of Advantage Media Group.

ADVANTAGE is a registered trademark and the Advantage colophon is a trademark of Advantage Media Group, Inc.

Printed in the United States of America.

ISBN: 978-159932-437-1
LCCN: 2014935282

This publication is designed to provide accurate and authoritative information in regard to the subject matter covered. It is sold with the understanding that the publisher is not engaged in rendering legal, accounting, or other professional services. If legal advice or other expert assistance is required, the services of a competent professional person should be sought.

Advantage Media Group is proud to be a part of the Tree Neutral® program. Tree Neutral offsets the number of trees consumed in the production and printing of this book by taking proactive steps such as planting trees in direct proportion to the number of trees used to print books. To learn more about Tree Neutral, please visit www.treeneutral.com. To learn more about Advantage's commitment to being a responsible steward of the environment, please visit www.advantagefamily.com/green

Advantage Media Group is a publisher of business, self-improvement, and professional development books and online learning. We help entrepreneurs, business leaders, and professionals share their Stories, Passion, and Knowledge to help others Learn & Grow. Do you have a manuscript or book idea that you would like us to consider for publishing? Please visit advantagefamily.com or call 1.866.775.1696.

DEDICATION

To Janie Robinson, RDH:

My personal cheerleader. Janie's passion for people, good work, teaching, and skills as a Master Communicator have allowed me to have the dental practice of my dreams and live my vision and mission in life. I am so grateful.

To Michael Horner and Emily Mitchmore, for loving me and my workaholic tendencies, and for giving me balance. To my many mentors and my patients. I truly stand on the shoulders of the giants who came before me.

With Love and Gratitude,

Randy (Dad)

ACKNOWLEDGEMENTS

Dr. Bill Blatchford and Blatchford Consulting for raising the standards in dentistry across the country by teaching dentists and their teams to respect the time and the value of the patients they serve.

Dr. Hugh Flax for Presidential Leadership in The American Academy of Cosmetic Dentistry and embracing diversity and fairness.

Dr. Arun Garg for founding the American Dental Implant Association and opening the world of dental implants for so many patients to enjoy. For his humanitarian efforts in the Dominican Republic to bring a high standard of dentistry to that country.

Sandy Roth for unselfish leadership in The American Academy of Cosmetic Dentistry and teaching thousands of dentists and their teams how important communication and organization are to our work.

Scott J Manning MBA for being the worlds foremost authority on business development and turning entrepreneurial passions into thriving enterprises for Professionals and Business Owners of all walks of life. He is a personal friend and advisor to Dr. Mitchmore. You can read his life, philosophies and receive valuable resources at www.MillionDollarMethods.com

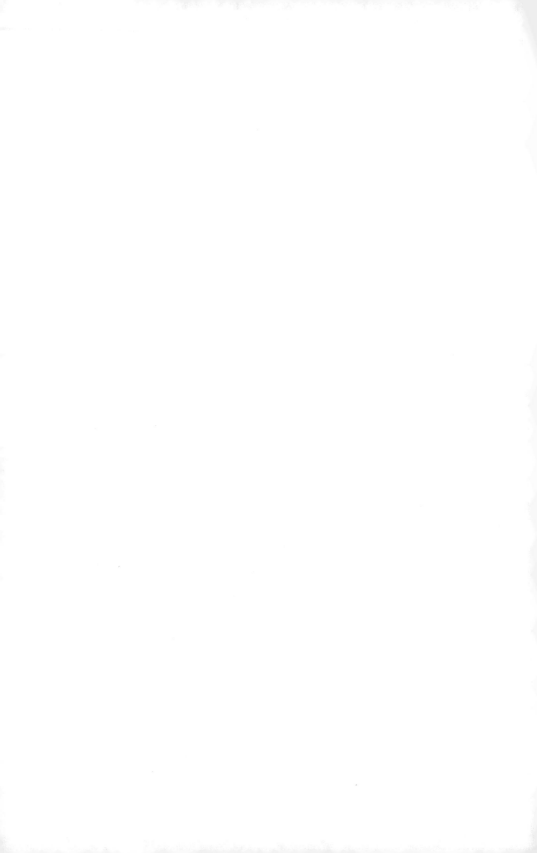

CONTENTS

INTRODUCTION

For most people these days, our healthcare system is more of a 'diseasecare' system. There is a huge amount of confusion out there about what to do to protect our health, as well as who to go to and how to pay for it.

I wrote this book to clear up this confusion where dentistry is concerned. It is a book for people who are seeking a good dentist, but it is also a book for other dentists. It is for dentists who are searching for ways to become what they always wanted to be, before they became trapped in the diseasecare model: Dentists who want to be mouth doctors instead of technicians fixing holes in teeth.

As for the patient who needs this book, you have probably been frustrated with dental care in the past, or had more than your fair share of bad dental experiences. After reading this, will learn that all dentists are not the same in their level of care, skill, and judgment. You will be able to self-evaluate the condition of your own mouth *and* the expertise of your dentist.

The key message you will learn here: Being confident that you have a good, healthy smile is a transformative feeling. The three action items I challenge you to accept to achieve that transformation are:

1. Don't settle for less than you want or deserve.
2. Listen to your gut intuition in selecting your dentist or the dentistry that you have done.
3. Realize that life is for Loving, Laughing, and Living. Don't put any of these things off. If the condition of your mouth or

smile is holding you back from reaping those rewards, what are you waiting for? If not today, when?

I was inspired to write this book because my patients have changed my life by and what they have taught me about Loving, Laughing and Living. In high school, I thought that I wanted to be a minister, and set my initial career path with that goal. For reasons you will soon read, I discovered that path was not right for me. However, I still consider myself a minister of sorts. I feel much the same way about my work that Marianne Williamson does when she writes in her own book *A Return to Love*:

> *You're in business to spread love. No matter what we do, we can make it our ministry. No matter what form our job or activity takes, the content is the same as everyone else's: We are here to minister to human hearts. If we talk to anyone, or see anyone, or even think of anyone, then we have the opportunity to bring more love into the universe. From a waitress to the head of a movie studio, from an elevator operator to the president of a nation, there is no one whose job is unimportant to God.*

My approach to dentistry is unique in that I am people centered rather than insurance centered. I am here to serve the needs of my dental patients, not the other way around. One way that I serve their needs is to forbid anyone who works in my office to lecture people, or make them feel bad in any way about the condition of their mouth or smile. Because my practice is focused on my patients' emotional needs as well as their dental needs, many of my patients are able to say that visiting my office is actually the first time they have enjoyed going to the dentist!

The experience of treating more than 75,000 people, coupled with my advanced training and belief that I am a perpetual student, has shaped my unique perspective on dentistry. I see too many dentists who chase after the latest gadget or technique rather than putting their focus on the patient's wants and desires. I feel badly for these dentists because they lack a clear mission and vision in their life, and in their work. Through this book, I would like to change that for them.

The legacy that I leave will be to raise the bar on what dentistry can do for the patient, as well as how dentists themselves can fulfill the true mission of dentistry: To transform lives through excellence, confidence, and caring.

CHAPTER 1

Why I Wrote This Book

I met Madonna on a blustery autumn day, after another dentist she'd seen advised her to come and see me.

A single mother raising three children, an ordained minister, and a professionally trained counselor, Madonna had more than her fair share of responsibility. This bright, highly educated 48-year-old woman was doing everything in her power to defy the odds against succeeding in life—and she had become convinced that her teeth were threatening to sink her prospects for making a better life for herself and her children.

Madonna was keenly aware of what it takes to succeed in life— both personally and as a businesswoman. Consequently, she saw in herself the hesitation and lack of self-confidence she strove to instill in the people who came to her for help. She knew it was important to look the part—to show by personal example that a well-kempt appearance invited trust and promoted cooperation. She felt strongly that meeting these goals started with a smile.

Madonna was right.

Smiling is one of the few universal communications that is instantly understood by every human on the planet. We smile even before we are born. Ultrasound technology shows that developing babies appear to smile while in the womb.

Smiling can make you a healthier person by reducing levels of stress-enhancing hormones, such as cortisol, adrenaline, and dopamine—while increasing the level of mood-enhancing hormones and reducing overall blood pressure.

It has been scientifically proven that smiling can actually make you look good in the eyes of others. A recent study at Penn State University found that when you smile, you don't only appear more likable and courteous, but that you actually appear to be more competent.

For these reasons and more, I agreed with Madonna. If she was hesitant to smile, her confidence would be diminished and she wouldn't be able to reach her full potential to help others. I easily recognized how important this was to her, since helping others is equally important to me.

During that first visit, we took a look at the dental reasons for Madonna's reluctance to smile. She gave me her concerns and I conducted a complete dental physical that included X-rays and diagnostic photographs. What I discovered during the time I spent with Madonna was that smiling—and laughter, and a passion for life—really did come naturally for her. The condition of her teeth had created a huge barrier for her to be her true, natural self.

Madonna was missing a front tooth. The rest of her teeth were significantly discolored due to age—fillings that used to be white were turning dark, and old metal fillings between the teeth were darker still.

She had previously been fitted with what's known as a "flipper," a fake tooth mounted on a piece of pink plastic that fits in the mouth and over the palate like an orthodontic retainer. A flipper looks like a fake tooth and functions at about 20 percent of a real tooth. The rest of Madonna's teeth were broken down, and none of them matched her personality. In fact, they actually inhibited her from fully smiling; she'd developed the habit of hiding her smile with her hand or lips. Ninety percent of communication is body language, and Madonna did not want her body language to convey that she might be hiding something and could not be trusted.

Together, Madonna and I reviewed the photographs of her mouth, discussing how it was possible to have a tooth permanently attached to her own teeth, and make them all whiter, straight, and beautiful at the same time. She was thrilled. She shared with me that she could not even imagine what it would be like to live without the constant fear that her flipper was going to break in public, creating the ultimate embarrassing and awkward moment. She couldn't imagine what it would be like to not hide her smile from people she really cared about, or not end every evening by reaching into her mouth, removing part of her smile, and putting in a bedside glass of water. The prospect of a life without such burdens, and of looking and feeling sexy and attractive to a potential mate, was a dream come true. Until we discussed how much it would cost.

Madonna was immediately deflated; her hopes were dashed. She said, "Oh, Dr. Mitchmore, I so badly want this. I've dreamed about this for so long. But with my healthcare expenses and raising children, I don't see any way that I could ever afford this. Even though this would make such a difference, I have to consider my priorities. My children come first. My car is totally undependable, and I have to pay for a new one before considering anything else. Thank you very much for your time; you have been very kind."

We parted respectfully—and I know both of us felt disappointed. I did not expect to see Madonna again.

A couple of months went by and Madonna called, asking to review her options again. She came in for another complimentary consultation. We sat together in my private office and looked at her photographs again, discussing the possibility of doing something less than ideal to save money. The second-best option was type of fake tooth that would definitely be better than her flipper, but wouldn't be permanently attached within her mouth; it would still need to be taken out to be cleaned and soaked.

Madonna knew in her heart that wasn't what she really wanted. She thanked me again for my time, and then went on her way.

This same scenario of coming in to talk about her options was repeated three times more! Each session ended the same way: Madonna knew what she wanted and deserved, but didn't think it would ever be possible.

Then one day my phone rang. "I have decided to get my smile back," Madonna said, "and I think I have found a way to pay for it. I want to start tomorrow!"

After doing some further research, Madonna had found a perfect yet inexpensive car. Unexpectedly, she now had the means to begin the process of repairing her smile. She confided in me that she really did not know exactly how she was going to pay for everything from start to finish. But she had conviction and trust that God would make some unknown things happen in her life and it would all work out.

Though I was truly delighted to hear the news, at the same time I shook my head in wonder at how she would ever come up with the remaining funds. I knew that it would be a huge sacrifice for her. Then again, I was hardly born with a silver spoon in my own mouth, and had started with almost nothing to build the state-of-the-art dental practice that had always been my dream. Life had taught me that, often, the biggest sacrifices yield the most amazing rewards. Madonna was soon to learn that lesson, too.

We got started right away. I first sculpted the design of her new smile out of white wax. A rubber mold was made from that design. The big day arrived: Madonna came in and received a highly effective local anesthetic, along with some sedation to calm her excitement and anxiety. I cleaned out her old fillings and cavities and prepared the teeth to receive a permanent bridge and porcelain veneers. The rubber mold was used to make temporary teeth, which she'd wear while the dental lab made her porcelain bridge and veneers. The next step was my favorite part of a long dental appointment: I sat Madonna upright, freshened up her face with a warm moist towel, and handed her a mirror to look at her new smile.

I think her heart stopped for a second. I know she was speechless for a few moments. Then a burst of tears, followed by the words, "Wow!" and, "Oh my God!"

Now that is why I am a dentist. *Together we shared the joy (and some very big, long hugs!).*

A few weeks later Madonna came back to slip off the temporary teeth and bond on the porcelain bridge and veneers. They looked even better! For the first time in 24 years, Madonna willingly smiled her widest and most genuine smile—and continued smiling as we took a large number of photographs of her new look. A large portrait of Madonna and that smile, which we took that day, now hangs in my office.

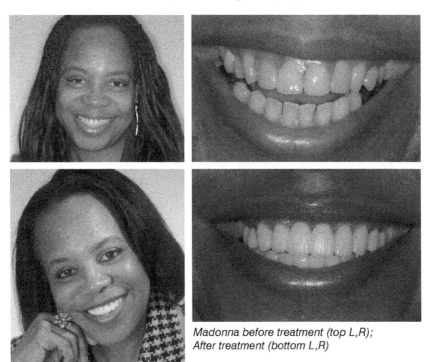

Madonna before treatment (top L,R);
After treatment (bottom L,R)

Madonna's story of transformation didn't end there. Shortly after her dental work was completed, she sent me the nicest thank-you note describing how her life was dramatically changing. All of a sudden, people were reacting to her differently. They were much more receptive to what she was saying, and much more outgoing toward her. Her work and income, as she put it, were "just exploding."

In reality, the people around Madonna hadn't changed—she had. Her confidence and inner beauty literally poured out, instead of being hidden or held in.

I look forward to those times that Madonna pops in the office unannounced just to say hello, since she's always smiling. Whenever I see her at fundraisers and other professional or social gatherings, we get to share a hug and a wink—because we know where she started, and where she is now.

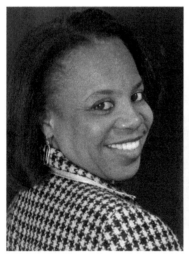 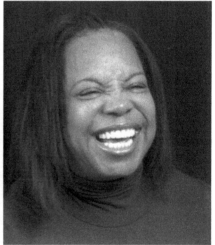

Madonna after treatment

To read more about Madonna's story and see full color before and after pictures of her now beautiful smile, visit **www.lifesmiles.us/reason**

I am Dr. Randy Mitchmore. By now, you're probably thinking this book is about being a dentist or going to the dentist. But it's not. This book is about discovery: Discovering that the power of a healthy smile, or lack thereof, can have everything to do with your confidence, performance, and where you go in life.

Madonna's life transformation is amazing, but it's not the only such story I could tell. In fact, I could easily fill several volumes with stories such as hers—of the transformations that people experience when they gain the confidence of a winning smile. I want you to know that if the condition of your mouth is preventing you from smiling, it's also preventing you from thriving—from living the life you deserve, and being the best you can be.

I have personally treated more than 75,000 private patients over a span of more than 25 years. I went to an outstanding liberal arts college and was trained in the largest medical center in the world. I had advanced dental training at several of the finest dental institutions on both sides of the country. I have achieved Master's honors in General Dentistry and Implant Dentistry. However, it is what my *patients* have taught me that has allowed me to get clear on my mission in life, and to live that mission. My mission in life is to create beauty and build people up. I live that mission by being a very good dentist.

I haven't always wanted to be a dentist. What I *have* always liked to do is build things, and make them nice or attractive. I have always been intrigued by how things are built or how they work. Basically, I feel the same about people. They've always intrigued me, and I'm pleased when I see them having a good time. Above all, I like making good things happen for people, and I appreciate those who've helped good things happen for me. I've always looked up to teachers, leaders, and all those who have fostered my love of learning.

Given my background, I should not have been as successful as I've turned out to be. I grew up living a childhood that looked nice, at least on the outside. My parents were the embodiment of the American Dream. They worked very hard—Dad went out to work while Mom raised five children. She watched for sales and collected S&H green stamps, had Tupperware parties, and bought a freezer to store bread and meat when it was on sale. On special occasions, we all went out to the Dinner Bell Cafeteria. Mom and Dad were Cubmasters and Den Leaders in Boy Scouts and we went to church every Sunday. And both my parents were very Victorian. No one in my family ever talked about sex, or even drank alcohol.

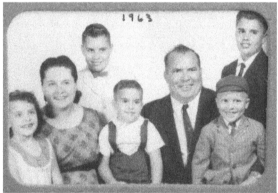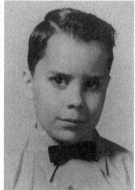

Early family photo; Dr. Mitchmore in the white jacket (L), Catholic grade school (R)

But as I grew up, I learned that this typical American Dream included ignoring a fair amount of bad stuff that went on behind the pretty appearance of my Leave It to Beaver family.

Of the four boys in the family, I was 'the good one.' I had this really mean older brother who was just the opposite. As I mentioned, I like to build things. He liked to tear things down. In work I've since done with The Mankind Project (a volunteer organization that trains men in communication, how to be better citizens and spouses, and basically what it means to be a man), I've learned that everyone has a shadow—a Darth Vader-like dark side that pulls at them. And to this day, I consider my older brother the root of my shadow. On one hand, I really like to build beautiful things and do good and serve people. But my dark side—the one that comes from my former pain, perhaps—sometimes pulls at me to tear things down.

My older brother called me 'Fatso,' and I called him 'Pimple-face' in a vain attempt to get back at him. He was physically violent—so violent that it scared me. I think it scared me into being the good boy. I didn't want to get involved in any of his 'bad' stuff. He and my father would get into fist-fights and shouting matches. My brother idolized Elvis Presley. He looked like him, and had the same Dippity-Do hairstyle. He was into motorcycles, guns, hanging out with the guys, smoking, and drinking—all the things associated with what we called a hoodlum back in those days. He ended up getting a girl pregnant and had to get married. They had two children, and he was so mean to her they finally divorced. But he had messed her up so badly that she ended up committing suicide. And he died, I think, of just plain meanness. In his 40s, he held the Harris County record for spending the most days in jail because he refused to pay child support. He said he'd rather go to jail. When he finally got out, he became a hermit, got cancer, and died.

Still, when I was a kid, my parents kept up appearances. Despite the violence inside my home, on the outside everything was fine. I always say my dad, bless his heart, was really a kind-hearted, sweet man. He worked hard, liked to play hard, and was good at sports. He never sought to be wealthy, never balanced a checkbook a day in his life, and was not concerned with his net worth as long as he could always pay his bills. He built the house we grew up in by adding another room himself each time a child was born.

My dad didn't really have a father figure of his own; he was 12 when his father died, so he had to go live with relatives in the summer. When he started having children, he knew it was important to be a father, but between building the house, working, and handling my older brother—gosh, he had his hands so full. When you divide your time between five children and one soaks up so much time, the time spent with your other kids gets spread thin. What we would call parenting skills certainly weren't taught back then. Probably the only 'learning resource' my dad had to draw from was watching TV.

Because I was so very different from anything else in his parenting experience, my father really didn't know how to handle me. I was sensitive and had no interest in sports. But he did his best—even though he liked sports and exposed me to them, he didn't demand that I participate. And he was truly God-fearing. He was close to being illiterate, so whatever the Bible said was literally written on stone tablets for him. He was always singing hymns out loud, and while he taught me how good it is to work hard and to fear God, he also taught me how good it is to laugh and play and sing.

As for my mother, she taught me to look out for myself, to save, and definitely to work hard. In her world, there was little time for play. Though she's softening a bit in her 80s, my mom was always critical of me when I was growing up. She would tell everyone else how proud she was *of* me, but she could never say it *to* me.

As a family, we kept our secrets well—right down to the big secret of the work my father did. When I was in school and it was time to tell everyone what your dad did to make a living, I had to say that he "had vending machines." That was a cover-up for the real truth. What he and my grandfather actually did was sell condoms out of vending machines. At that time, the word 'condom' was censored from TV and movies because it was considered unspeakably nasty, but my dad was selling them out of machines in the restrooms of gas stations, nightclubs, and strip-tease parlors. You put in a quarter and turned the crank, and out came something that nobody talked about.

So I grew up with the false notion that it was okay to cover up your inner workings when it was counter to the public norm. It was easier and better than having to explain things. After all, no real harm was done. You weren't exactly telling lies; they were just 'little white lies.' Those were okay—after all, they didn't do any real harm.

Later, I learned of the incredible harm that such secrets and lies could do—and, in fact, did do in my life. But I don't lay blame at my family's door, and I don't bear anger or bitterness toward them. I'm not that type of person; I don't hold anger or grudges for very long. I just view people as they are and let it go. Besides, I grew up learning many truly valuable lessons, and being fortunate in many ways. Those life lessons serve me today with my work and the patients who come to me.

CHAPTER 2

Is Dental Neglect Your Dirty Little Secret? It's Never Too Late to Set Yourself Free

Nune never feared visiting the dentist as a child. "I actually found it to be a positive experience," he says.

That changed during his adult years. After several unpleasant experiences, Nune put off dental maintenance for so long that his dental health reached a critical point. He had gotten into a cycle I often see: Nune knew he had serious problems, he knew that the news wouldn't be good, and he knew that seeing a dentist again would cause him more pain—psychologically and physically. So he simply kept procrastinating.

"Why bother?"

Why bother, indeed.

Unfortunately, going to see the dentist or a doctor usually isn't fun. Often, a painful procedure is involved. I'm referring to psychological pain: the discomfort of being led to feel that those who are treating you just don't care.

There are a multitude of reasons why our healthcare system seems to have lost the connection to empathy. Some of those reasons may have credence, but I'm not here to argue their validity. I'm here to say that ultimately, if you are unwell you have to overcome that lack of empathy.

You have to rise above uncaring, closed-circuit thinking and take responsibility for driving yourself back to good health. You have to overcome your fear—and, as they say, the first step to overcoming your fear is to look it in the face.

That's precisely what Nune did, albeit a bit belatedly. By the time he came to see me, he had a serious oral infection that had lead to significant bone loss in his jaw. His teeth were loose, and before things got better he would actually lose all of his teeth. The news was crushing to Nune. He knew that the pain and expense of treating his dental problems could very well have been prevented if he had only acted sooner—if he had only overcome his reluctance to seek help.

We're humans. We do that. We put off what we don't want to do. As a result, we feel guilty, or embarrassed. And then we do something worse: We tell ourselves that we deserve the bad stuff that happens because it's all our fault. And often, we hide behind those feelings of guilt and self-punishment. If we do only the slightest bit of self-assessment, though, we see the truth.

Nune saw it. "I had become very self-conscious about smiling for photos," he said. "It was impacting my life. I was only hurting myself by not doing anything."

When you shut off your smile, you deactivate one of the main avenues of communicating your sociability. You're sending subtle messages to those around you that you're not amenable to interaction, either socially or professionally. It may take a while to notice, but ultimately you will notice it. Friends and coworkers will seem distant.

The human smile is an invitation to others. The lack of it means, "Stay away."

After I consulted with Nune, he decided that dental implants would be his course of action. Surgery would be required to remove his teeth, including grafts for his damaged and infected jawbone. It was a long process, that journey back to good health. My top priority was to make his journey from fear about the process to welcoming the changes that lie ahead as short as possible. That's important—VERY important.

I can't do my job without my patients' participation. I needed Nune to be a willing player in his recovery, which meant he had to give himself permission to stop feeling guilty about the situation he had created for himself. That started with making sure he never had a reason to feel uncomfortable when he was in my office. It started me with asking him, "Nune, how can I help you face your fear?"

Of course, Nune's physical health was of top priority throughout his journey. At one of his routine post-op visits he asked if he might need an antibiotic because he was not feeling well. He had lost weight and developed a cough, and wondered if the grafts had become infected and affected his lungs. I carefully examined Nune's mouth and assessed his overall physical status. I then looked him in the eye and said, "Nune, removing the bad teeth and having the implants would not cause this kind of weight loss and cough. I can see that you are really sick and you need to get to a physician right away." I was right; Nune was diagnosed with a very serious illness. Thankfully, he listened to me, and has responded very well to treatment. His life was transformed because he developed trust in me, and confidence in the fact that he was worthy of being healthy.

Today, Nune will tell you that he's well on his way to being the healthiest he's ever been in his life. He'll also gladly tell you that his physical health is inextricably tied to his emotional well-being. "I'm smiling more than ever," Nune says. And he's reaping the rewards from it.

Nune re-hung the 'Welcome' sign in his life when he regained his smile.

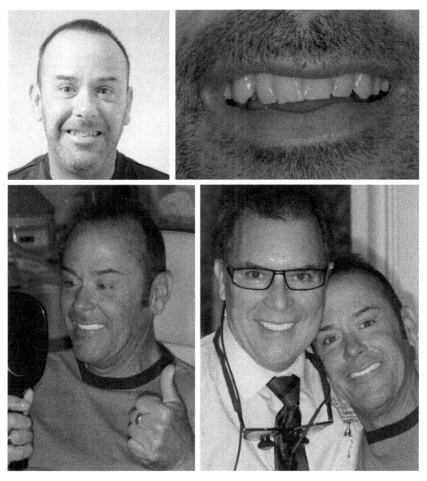

Nune before treatment (top L,R); After treatment (bottom L,R)

To read more about Nune's story and to discover how you too can set yourself free with a healthy and beautiful smile visit **www.lifesmiles.us/ freedom.**

The thought of going to the dentist conjures up a familiar scenario in most people's minds: You go in and the dentist looks in your mouth. Depending on what he or she sees, you may get a lecture about all the mistakes you've made. Then you'll get told what you need, and you're supposed to nod your head and say, "Yes, yes. That's what I'll do." You probably feel shamed.

If that's been your experience, I apologize. A lot of people's negative thoughts about going to the dentist stem from past experiences; I want to change their old perceptions and create a new experience. So I spend a lot of time telling my patients, "I have to apologize for my profession. I have to apologize for dentists letting you down." I don't lecture. I'm not into playing the shame and blame game. I do not judge. And if there's one phrase I strictly prohibit anyone in my office from using, it's, "This is what you need to do."

I don't tell patents what they should do. I ask them, "What do you want?" It's a totally different way of interacting with people. I don't approach dentistry as the all-seeing, all-knowing doctor telling people what they need, because it's not about *me*. It's about *you*. My role as a dentist is to provide you with the information you need to make your own decisions, to choose the treatments that you feel are best for you. Once you make that choice, I can then use my expertise to give you the very best results.

Before we can talk about what you really want, however, you need to give yourself permission to go after it. I've found that many people have trouble with that—they don't give themselves permission to get what they really want, and what they really deserve. One of the things I think you deserve is enjoying the gift of good health. That's what general dentistry is all about: Keeping your teeth and gums healthy, because there's an intimate connection between your *oral* health and your *overall* health.

Part of that health connection is psychological. I can't tell you how many times I've seen transformations in patients who've been embarrassed about their appearance—we fix their smile and they come back a year later totally transformed. Their confidence has doubled. Many times, they can actually dollarize the difference, since many have told me that their income has more than doubled, too.

But the health connection that general dentistry is primarily devoted to is the preservation of, and improvement in, your physical health. The mouth really is a window to the inside of the body. It reveals a lot of unhealthy disease issues that can be going on in the rest of your body.

Take periodontal or gum disease, for example. Sure, it causes oral concerns like bad breath and tooth loss. But this condition is not isolated to the mouth. In fact, scientists believe it may be linked to more than 200 other diseases. It causes inflammation in the body that can be measured in the blood by *C–reactive protein* tests. If your gums bleed, it's a sure sign that infection is present—and I can promise you that along with that infection there is inflammation. That inflammation in your gums is causing inflammation of the blood vessels in and around your heart. This promotes arterial plaque—the buildup of fatty deposits in your arteries. And that can make you really sick. It can cause a heart attack or stroke.

Some of the other connections scientists have uncovered between gum disease and whole-body health: Breast, mouth, throat, kidney, pancreatic, and brain cancers have all been linked to gum disease. In diabetics, gum disease can impact insulin sensitivity and lead to unhealthy blood sugar levels. Bacteria originating from the teeth and gums may cause lung infections or aggravate pre-existing respiratory conditions. Gum inflammation may also be a major player in chronic health concerns besides heart disease, such as rheumatoid arthritis and Alzheimer's disease.

The other big concerns in general dentistry are cavities and tooth loss, of course. Tooth decay can cause teeth to become infected. Sometimes, people develop acute, rapid-onset infections that cause an unbelievable amount of pain. Pain is a powerful motivator, so that brings them running to the dentist faster than anything else. But I've also seen many cases in which someone had a 'little' toothache that they kind of ignored, hoping it would go away. The next day, and the day after that, it got worse—and by the fourth day, that someone woke up with a face so swollen it was shocking. Both of these situations can be truly life threatening. Obviously, they're situations we want to avoid.

By going in for regular dental care, you can prevent such painful problems. You can also prevent the tooth loss that goes hand in hand with decay and gum disease. There's a scientific study that just showed a strong relationship between how many teeth people have and what their lifespan is. In general, the number of teeth a person loses over his or her life is a marker of the disease processes going on. The bottom line: As you lose more teeth, your lifespan gets shorter. If you really want to not just live longer, but be healthier and feel better *as* you live longer, do what has to be done to get your teeth and gums healthy.

Keeping your teeth not only means you may live longer, but it also means you feel good longer. Case in point: Tooth loss impacts your chewing ability, and if you're not chewing properly, you're not going to have proper digestion. You may not even be eating the foods you should, which means you'll sacrifice nutrition. You'll sacrifice being as healthy as you can be, and feeling as wonderful as you could feel.

Why Not Wait?

Some people whose dental problems have developed over the years will get to the point where they feel their problems are so monumental, and will cost so much money to fix, that they give up entirely. They develop an attitude of, "Well, since there's no hope of fixing my teeth, there's no sense in really doing anything. I'll just get dentures later."

The reality is that modern dentistry *can* work modern miracles, but dentures are artificial replacements of body parts. And as good a dentist as I am, even I can't replace a real body part with an artificial one and tell you it's just as good. Let me ask you: If you injured your thumb and it got pretty mangled, would your first impulse be to amputate your thumb, or even your whole arm? Would you say, "Well, I'll just let it get worse; they can take the whole arm off and just give me an artificial one"? I doubt it, because you know that an artificial arm might look something like a real arm, and give you some capabilities. But it's not going to function like your old arm did.

Artificial teeth are the same way. I advise people to think long and hard before having a tooth amputated. However, if a tooth is badly infected or has gangrene (yes, gangrene), or is cracked in two, there is no debate—it must be removed, and the sooner the better. Otherwise it can make your whole body sick. But artificial teeth are still artificial body parts. If someone gets dentures, their chewing ability is reduced by about 70 percent. There is also the discomfort of denture irritation, and the hassle of having to replace them every five or 10 years because they wear out and get stinky.

Up to now, most dentures and partials have been made out of acrylic. Acrylic is porous. Bacteria in our mouths love to have warm, dark, moist places thrive in, and porous materials give them such places. That is why dentures can really stink. Fungus likes porous acrylic too, so when it's pressed against the gums, the gums get inflamed and infected and make you sick.

There are also cosmetic considerations, many of which we'll get into later. I see patients who have porcelain crowns that were made with the old technology, meaning they're fused to a silver-colored metal. These frequently look dark grey at the gumline. The silver metal often is a base metal much like cheap costume jewelry is made from, and if it touches the gums, the gums react to it in a negative way.

Don't get me wrong—today, there are ways we can drastically reduce those artificial body-part problems. In fact, much of my practice is devoted to high-end tooth restoration techniques. Instead of porous acrylic, I can use milled zirconium. It's more durable and bacteria-resistant. For crowns, I use newer technology that is all porcelain. There is no caustic metal in it. My point is that it's far superior to save your natural teeth if we can. Technology is wonderful, and we can do some really wonderful things for people, but artificial teeth still aren't as good as the real thing.

As I said earlier, I think you deserve the best, and I want to give it to you. So I'd prefer to save the teeth you have, and restore your mouth to a healthy state. You'd be surprised at how many times that can be done. And you'd probably be surprised at how comfortably I can do it.

CHAPTER THREE

The Complete Dental Physical: A Cornerstone of the Care You Deserve

Being a celebrity often means setting aside things you want to do for things you have to do. Rick Davis had done just that regarding his smile. He certainly had good reason to put off dental care. He was constantly on the go as a singer with the Grammy Award-winning Texas Swing band Asleep At The Wheel. And when he wasn't performing, Rick was back at home in Livingston caring for his elderly mother. So when the moment came to focus a little bit of attention on himself, Rick decided it was time for his smile to take center stage. After all, as a performer, he was keenly aware that his appearance was part of what brought people to see Asleep At The Wheel perform. But Rick had a particular concern that set him apart from many other patients: He was worried that any major changes made to the shape of his teeth, or how his teeth and lips came together, might affect his singing ability. And when you make your living with your voice, that's certainly something you don't want to mess with!

Rick's search for a professional with the expertise to address his unique concern led him from California all the way to Houston, Texas. Here, he ultimately selected me to help him with a major dental makeover.

A large corporate dental implant chain had suggested removing all of Rick's teeth and replacing them with implants. "I know I need my teeth fixed up," he said to me, "but that seems pretty drastic." It is, and unfortunately it is often the standard approach that corporate dental implant chains take. I don't approach things the same way. There is no cookie-cutter answer, because I feel each person is unique.

I shared Rick's concern that such a major change really could impact how he sang. Speaking (and in this case, singing) properly has a great deal to do with the positioning of the teeth between the lips and the tongue. We have all heard someone with bad dentures lisp or whistle when they talk, which is the result of the tip of the tongue failing to make a seal against the teeth. In order to make a good "E" sound, the lower teeth have to come ever so close to the edges of the top teeth without banging in to them. A good "F" or "V" sound requires the correct position of the top teeth relative to the lower lip.

For Rick, the best solution was far less drastic than what he had been told. It involved keeping many of his natural teeth and augmenting them with dental implants only where truly necessary. I made models of Rick's own teeth and jaws. I used these models to design his new smile, sculpting broken-down teeth back to their original shape and filling in areas of missing teeth to follow the original contours of his smile. I then made silicone molds of the sculpted teeth.

Nevertheless, it was a lot of work—but that work was made easier for Rick by using IV Sedation. As he slipped into the dental chair, he was pampered with booties on his feet, a cozy blanket, and headphones that allowed him to listen to the kind of music he liked. We started an IV, and a computer monitor was connected to track vital signs for safety. Then I administered the sedation drugs that I affectionately refer to as "Hugs and Kisses." Within minutes, Rick was in a state of bliss, and my team and I went to work. By the end of the morning, we'd done several proce-

dures in a matter of hours: Rick's teeth and gums were deep-cleaned, his broken-down teeth had been restored, implants were placed only where needed, and his new temporary teeth placed. When it was time to reveal his new look that morning, I handed him a mirror and the first words out of his mouth were my favorites: "Wow, I love it!"

As many patients do, he wanted to express his gratitude for the transformation in his life. So at one of his follow-up appointments, he brought his guitar and sang a few songs for us while sitting in the dental chair!

The treatment Rick underwent in my office was far less invasive than his initial 'chain dentist' had pitched—which meant it cost less, as well. Even more importantly, Rick retained the shape of his mouth and, therefore, the uniqueness of his voice. The moral to this story, I think, is that what we are given by heredity shapes our lives. Rick made the decision that was right for him, and I was glad to help him regain a beautiful smile and retain the singing career he loved.

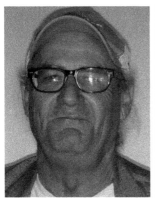
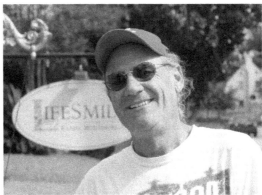

Rick before treatment (top L,R); After treatment with Dr. Mitchmore (bottom R)

To read more about Rick's story and to discover the transformational power of Prettau dental implants visit **www.lifesmiles.us/ completecare**

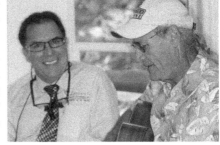

Making the decisions that are right for you can literally change the course of your life. That's something I've not only seen in my practice, but also learned in my own life. As I've already mentioned, I didn't always want to be a dentist. In fact, I initially studied to become a Methodist minister. I studied and received a license to preach from The United Methodist Church before graduating high school, then entered college at Southwestern University in Georgetown, Texas.

What lessons in humility I learned there! It was a private liberal arts college for rich kids, but I was there on an academic and work scholarship. When I wasn't studying, I was in the cafeteria busing tables, washing dishes, and mopping up after the rich kids while they went outside and played. That was hard to take, since my eyes had just been opened to the fact that there was life *outside* of work! Harder still was the fact that I was having trouble cutting it academically. At the time, the natural path to becoming a minister meant majoring and minoring in English and Religion, so I did that my first year. Through advanced placement, I skipped the typical freshman courses and was taking upper level courses. I struggled with English literature in translation. I was just lost as could be.

I soon realized I could no longer go in a direction where I was copying someone else. I had to do what *I* wanted to do.

After my first dreadful year at Southwestern, I decided to test the waters in the Science Department by going to summer school at The University of Houston. I LOVED science, and excelled at it. So I went back to Southwestern as a Science major and found myself. My best friend and roommate, Dod Moore, and I decided to become dentists. Dod didn't want to be a physician like his father; I had a distant uncle who was a dentist with what appeared to be a good life. In dentistry, I knew I could exercise my love of science and my love of service to others at the same time. A decision was made. We both finished our college work in only three years and we both were accepted to The University of Texas Dental Branch in Houston.

My dream had come true, but I had no idea how to pay for it. So I went back to work. I took a position at the old V.A. Hospital in Houston—in exchange for drawing blood on the T.B. ward at 5:30 every morning, I could eat in the hospital cafeteria, and live in a concrete dormitory that had a common bathroom and no air conditioning. I rode a bicycle to dental school, and then worked in the Methodist Hospital next door until 11 p.m. It was a nightmare—I lost 30 pounds that first year! But the lessons in hard work I'd learned from my mother served me very

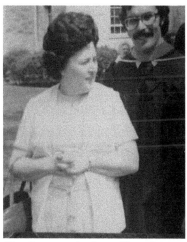

At college graduation with mother

well, as did the experience I gained. My work in the blood bank and the pathology lab, which involved drawing blood from patients with all kinds of medical problems, taught me a great deal about medicine that my dental school classmates did not learn in the lecture halls. This knowledge and experience would come to serve me well in my dental career—especially when I took the large leap to be certified and licensed to give IV Sedation. Very few dentists are able to make the sacrifices needed to learn and pass the rigorous higher requirements for licensure. Pursuing my dreams was definitely the right decision.

When it comes to making the right personal dental decisions, the first thing you need to know is where your oral health stands now. That means at your first appointment, I have to find out what you want and where you are now by gathering information in a comprehensive way.

My staff and I use an 18-point checklist to make sure we gather all the information needed. I'll admit to asking a lot of questions, and I want you to be as honest with me as I am with you. Some of the things we do are probably pretty familiar to you if you've visited a dentist within five to 10 years, but others go way beyond the usual scope. We'll find out what your major concerns are, and what brought you to us for dental care. We'll take your blood pressure and heart rate, and get some details on your medical history. And we'll take very detailed close up photographs and x-rays—though those x-rays may be a far cry from the ones you've had in the past.

The type of x-rays I use are digital x-rays. Technically, they're conventional X-rays but they aren't the tradition "film" type. Digital x-rays expose the patient to 90 percent less radiation than old film x-rays do; plus, they provide a tremendous improvement in terms of image clarity. They're also instant. In the past, the patient would have to wait up to an hour after an X-ray was taken for images to be developed. With digitals, images are ready in one to two seconds. They're much healthier for the patient, much better for the planet, and much more helpful to me, your dentist.

In some cases, I also use 3D X-rays as a diagnostic tool. With these, I can see aspects of the mouth that are totally impossible to see with either the naked eye or other dental instruments. In effect, they allow me to do "exploratory surgery" within the mouth without cutting it open to look into it. With 3D x-rays, I can identify cracks in teeth, changes in bone, and abscesses that other types of x-rays won't spot. I can literally look inside the jaws and the roots of the teeth. The technology is so incredible that I use it when planning implant surgery, to generate precise models of the implants themselves. I also use it when doing implant surgery, as it allows me to place implants without even making an incision.

Other aspects of your initial exam include checking your saliva flow and pH acid level [see 'Why Lube Is a Must'] and screening for TMD [see Chapter Five]. We'll also look for any signs of oral cancer—something I believe that every dentist should do at every patient's checkup. Oral cancer is now more common than cervical cancer, and though it can be very disfiguring, it has a very high cure rate when caught early. My practice uses special lights to detect it more easily, as well as patient-friendly 'brush biopsies' instead of scalpels to get samples of suspicious tissue that are sent out for tests. From start to finish, your initial appointment will last about an hour and a half. There aren't very many dentists who are that thorough; the vast majority will take five or 10 minutes to do an examination. That's hardly enough time for me to get to know you, or get to know your mouth. I believe that you deserve my time and attention, so that's what you get.

When your first appointment is over, we'll schedule your next one. That's your treatment conference, where the information we've gathered will be put to good use. You will discover why the close-up photographs become diagnostic tools.

At the treatment conference, we sit elbow-to-elbow to discuss all of the clinical and diagnostic data that has been collected, and merge it with what you tell me you want. The process is much like a puzzle—all the information we both need is there, we just have to figure out how to fit it together. We will look at your actual photographs and you will be very involved in deciding exactly what is to be done. Together, we will develop a detailed plan of action for you. This time together is extremely important to make sure your plan is clear and that it meets your goals and expectations. A thorough conference prevents disappointment, and paves the way for a successful and happy relationship.

> ### *Every minute spent in planning*
> ### *saves two in execution.*
>
> **—Henry Kaiser,** Kaiser Aluminum and Health Foundation

CHAPTER FOUR

Gums of Steel: Resting Easy About Gum Disease

The path that people take to find me is always interesting. Many come by word of mouth. Some come in because they drive by and see the unique and attractive building or Brutus, the wrapped Smart Car, out front. Still others will send their spouse in as a guinea pig to make sure my practice is a good, safe place.

No matter what path new patients take to find me, most of them make an initial appointment knowing that they have some unattended dental problem, but uncertain about how to start the resolution process. They want to proceed with caution, to 'put their toe in the water' first. The typical way they put their toe in the water is to call and say, "I want to have my teeth cleaned and checked."

Of course, all new patients fill out information forms, but in my practice I keep them as short as possible. I don't like filling out forms, and experience has taught me that a majority of people share my view. Experience has also taught me that most people live in denial of signs of health issues, and/or do not feel it is important to reveal their health problems to a dentist. So when I first examine a new patient, part of my job is to be a sleuth—a Sherlock Holmes, if you will. That's why my new patient dental physical will often take up to 90 minutes. I have to gather tons of data and search for clues to determine what the existing dental problems are and what may be causing those problems. In addition, I have to work with the patient to find out what his or her concerns and wants are, and a get a sense of what is wanted or expected in the future.

Norma's story illustrates the importance of this multi-faceted 'detective' approach. Norma's grown son came to me first. He had been referred by his own dentist, who does not offer the advanced dental procedures that I do. Once Norma's son had a good experience at my practice and told his mom about us, Norma decided it was her turn.

My Sherlock Holmes time with her was intense. I found that most every tooth in her mouth had either a filling, a root canal, a crown— or all three! There were a lot of cavities. Norma's mouth was very dry with little saliva flow, and her saliva was acidic. The gums had an odor, and they were cyanotic or purple in color where porcelain fused to metal crowns encroached into the gums. She had bad breath and yellow spots in her eyes. I also observed that the vertical length of the lower third of her face had collapsed, making her look much older than her years.

Norma's dental physical didn't end with her mouth, however. None of my dental physicals do.

I noted that her posture was extremely poor. One shoulder dipped one way, the pelvis dipped the other, and her head dipped the opposite way to compensate—carried forward of the shoulders. She told me she frequently had headaches, and the muscles of her jaws were tender to the touch. Just lying in the dental chair (tilted back slightly to check her gums for disease) made her dizzy.

Norma was very sick, and she knew it. Indeed, it turned out that she had been to a number of physicians and was seeking out multiple alternative health providers—including a cranio-sacral chiropractor, an acupuncturist, and a nutritionist. Adding to her burden was the fact *that Norma hated going to the dentist. I really couldn't blame her—she'd obviously had quite a lot of prior dentistry done, much of it painful.*

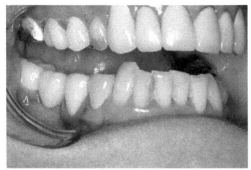

Norma's gums before treatment

Clearly, there was much that needed to be done. But first I had to ask a lot of questions to determine what was causing her problems—and then ask more questions to determine how much we could accomplish for Norma based on her budget. Each and every question is crucial. If we don't delve fully into the causes of all problems and find solutions to them, history will indeed repeat itself.

My dental team and I came up with a list of Norma's problems and their probable causes. Believe it or not, Norma's dry mouth topped the list of concerns. Saliva is so important to maintaining health of the teeth that Norma's crowns and filling were failing from a lack of it. Her gums were diseased from the combination of several factors: dry mouth, base-metal allergies to crowns buried in her gums, rotten cavity-filled teeth, and bacterial infection that her weak immune system was not fighting very well.

Norma's muscle spasms, posture issues, headaches, and dizziness were related to her mouth, as well. They were caused by a bad bite. You might ask, "With all of the crowns that she'd had done, how could she have a bad bite?" My answer: Easily. I see it all the time.

Norma had so many different kinds of crowns and fillings in her mouth done over the years that it literally looked like a patchwork quilt.

This happens often—one dentist may do a crown or two without perfecting the bite. The patient feels that the bite is off a tiny bit, but figures she has to "get used to it." A couple of years later, a move across the country to another city means finding another dentist. A problem comes up and another crown and a root canal are done. The bite drifts off center just a bit more, and the patient figures she will "get used to it" just like she did before. (I also find that in situations like this the reason the nerve died in some teeth—thus causing a need for a root canal—is because of a bad bite. The teeth literally got pounded to death!)

Twenty-two crowns later, you can see where Norma might be. We decided to start with the foundation—the gums and bone around the teeth. She had to go through our Gums of Steel program. Under the comfort of IV Sedation, Norma had a deep cleaning. This removed the crusty hard deposits from the roots of the teeth, eliminating a major source of destructive bacteria. Then she started a basic regimen that involved steering clear of sugary mints such as Altoids, raising the pH of her saliva with products and foods containing Xylitol, vigilantly removing the daily biofilm that grows on the teeth, and using some cool tools to get between the teeth without floss.

Norma responded extremely well to the Gums of Steel program, and within a week she could taste and feel the difference it made in her mouth. She was then ready to discuss the next step: Some of her teeth were so damaged they had to be removed. In fact, she was faced with needing a complete overhaul—what is commonly called a 'full mouth restoration.'

Norma did not want any bridges. (Bridges involve fitting the teeth on both sides of a missing tooth with crowns, then gluing the bridge itself to those crowns to cover the gap in between). She knew that bridges would be hard to clean, which would increase the risk of further cavities. She also did not want anything that was removable, so full or partial dentures were out. There was a lot to think about, and it took Norma two months of wrestling about how much could be done in a session, and how she could budget for it. You see, my fee for doing the work is tied to how much is done at any one time.

That may sound strange at first, but people are not paying me for a 'crown.' They are actually paying for my time, expertise, judgment, care, quality of materials used, and my advanced skill level. My charges are much like those of a lawyer who charges an hourly rate, plus incidental expenses, such as copies, research expenses, etc. Frankly, not all lawyers are the same; some are much better than others. The better ones charge a higher rate because they are more successful in helping you—and they usually save you money in the long run. Many patients have discovered the hard way that not all dentists are the same, either. I do not charge one specific fee for a crown or veneer and just multiply that by the amount of veneers that need to be done. I believe in passing along cost savings to the patient when I can. If I do one crown, it involves the same appointment process, preparation of the room and all sterile supplies, and follow-up that I use when doing 10 crowns at a time. Yes, the time and lab bill are more for the 10-crown visit – but not 10 times more. So I can pass those cost savings to the patient.

Grouping work together in sessions is cost effective for both my patients and me. It was also the ideal situation for Norma, especially with her level of anxiety and dread of dental work. She opted to have all her dental work done at one time.

It took several months of work re-establishing a bite that was harmonious with her joints and muscles, and where her teeth could fit together comfortably. This is called NeuroMuscular Dentistry. Its guiding principle is to establish harmony with the joints and muscles of the jaw. Most dentists take an opposite approach: They let the way teeth currently interdigitate, or bite together, dictate where they build the bite for the next crown, even when the way the currently interdigitate is not in harmony. Why? Because it is easier that way!

True, the way we re-established a healthy bite for Norma wasn't exactly easy. It involved testing her new bite with an orthotic, much like some people place an orthotic in their shoe to make up for one leg being shorter than the other. The patient wears the orthotic bonded to the teeth for one to three months or more. During this time, the new bite that I build is tested with computer readings of the jaw muscles (EMGs) to verify that we have it right.

I do it the hard way because it's the better way. As Norma's case illustrates, the negative consequences of a bad bite can be far reaching— and the results of correcting the situation are more than worth the effort. The orthotic worked wonders for Norma. Her muscle symptoms and headaches began to clear up and go away! What's more, her gums were again healthy. She was ready for the next stage.

Digital scans of her teeth were made. Norma appreciated that because she was used to having gooey rubber impressions made for her crowns, which always made her sick from gagging. Resin models of her teeth were made from those digital scans; then her new teeth were sculpted in white wax in preparation for her big day.

An hour before her appointment, she donned comfortable clothes and took a sedative that I prescribed for her. Her husband drove her to the office. Once she was comfortable in the dental chair, we removed her shoes and replaced them with nice warm booties. We also warmed a 'Huggie' in the microwave and wrapped that over her neck and shoulders. (Huggies are made by my 92-year-old patient, Robbie. She creates a beautiful form-fitting collar that is filled with aromatic herbs and spices. My patients find it incredibly effective at helping them relax.)

Next, we connected Norma to an EKG, blood pressure cuff, and a pulse oximeter to monitor her vital signs during her procedures. An

IV was started and I delivered the sedation drugs that I call "Hugs and Kisses." Within minutes, Norma was in a state of bliss and the real work of transformation could begin.

Norma's four severely damaged teeth were removed and dental implants were put in their place. Then all of her old crowns and fillings were removed, and all of her cavities were cleaned out and sealed. Finally, all of the teeth were then gently prepared and shaped to receive metal-free porcelain crowns and veneers. Temporary crowns and veneers were made from the molds I had previously sculpted out of wax.

The 'reveal' took place when Norma's sedation wore off. She held up a mirror to look at her new smile, and that's when she realized the change affected far more than her teeth. She actually had an overall much younger look because vertical length had been restored to her face. In effect, she'd gotten a dental facelift.

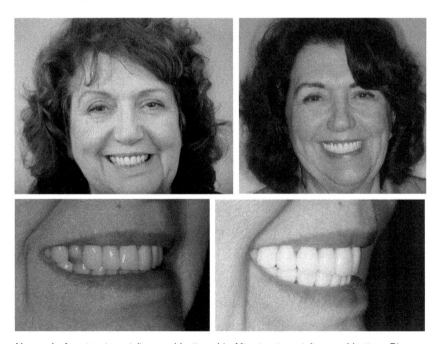

Norma before treatment (top and bottom L); After treatment (top and bottom R)

What's more, she'd gotten a new lease on life, through incredible improvements in her health. Her mouth had been literally making her sick. Even worse, the positioning of her teeth and jaws were stealing her youth and trapping her in a shadowy world of constant headaches and dizziness. So much of Norma's physical ailments were directly related to the condition of her teeth that by resolving her dental problems, she gained many improvements in her health. Her experience illustrates one of the things I love most about being a dentist—and one of the most powerful things I've learned about life. It's not always easy to tackle an issue we've struggled with for years, but when we do, we're rewarded in more ways that we ever dreamed.

To read more about Norma's story and to discover how a healthy mouth creates a healthier life visit **www.lifesmiles.us/healthygums.**

Before I graduated from dental school, I got married to the only woman I dated in college. I met her after my first year of working in the cafeteria. By then, I was working in the library and she came in to check out a book. She looked kind of cute, pretty and soft. She was friendly, and I needed a date soon for a party. I called her up and asked her to go and she said yes.

I was accepted into dental school a year early, and when she graduated from Southwestern she followed me to Houston. At that time, I was going with the flow of society, and of life. Everything was moving pretty fast, and my best friend was dating a girl and getting married, so I pretty much followed suit. Millie was bright, fun, and a talented and creative artist, and I loved her family. I really fell in love with her family as much I did with her. Marrying her just seemed like the next logical step in building my own American Dream—of living the good life with a nice home and 2.2 children and two cars in the garage.

After we married, life moved even faster. I graduated early and purchased a used building from my distant uncle, the dentist, the following week. We moved to a very small country town called Cleveland, in the Piney Woods of East Texas. I hung my shingle out as the new dentist in town, and did all the right things. I worked very hard and joined all of the service organizations. The townspeople welcomed my devotion to the betterment of the community, since most of the other young doctors in the area chose to live in a nice suburb of Houston and commute to this sawmill town. I was elected three different times to serve as a City Councilman, and my practice grew quickly. In dentistry, I'd truly found my calling—I was (and still am!) in love with the profession, and the chance it gave me to help other people. And I enjoyed the lifestyle it provided. I had nice cars, a custom home, and travelled—across the country, to Europe, to Canada, and to Mexico. I ate at fine restaurants, went scuba diving, and played golf.

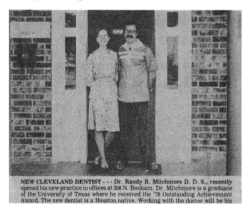

NEW CLEVELAND DENTIST - - - Dr. Randy R. Mitchmore D. D. S., recently opened his new practice in offices at 206 N. Bonham. Dr. Mitchmore is a graduate of the University of Texas where he received the '78 Outstanding Achievement Award. The new dentist is a Houston native. Working with the doctor will be his

First dental office

On the outside, I was the definition of success. But on the inside, I was conflicted and confused in my marriage.

I continued my dental education at the finest dental institute in the world, traveling from Texas to Key Biscayne, Florida, a couple of times each year. There, I was taught about the importance of balance between work and play, love and worship. I was schooled in principals of dentistry that said know yourself, know your patient, know your work, and apply your knowledge. That's where I really started becoming more aware. I was totally out of balance. I was struggling with 'know yourself.' And in that struggle, I was also struggling with the balance between 'know yourself' and 'know your patient.' The conflict in my personal life became a drag on my professional performance—and given my love for dentistry, that was immensely painful for me.

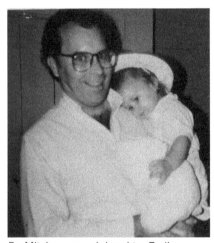

Dr. Mitchmore and daughter Emily

Then, after 14 years of marriage, my beautiful daughter Emily was born. She was a blessing, a gift. I grabbed onto being a parent. It provided another diversion from facing my own feelings of discontent. I loved my daughter intensely, and I loved the whole idea of having a family. I wanted to have the house in the country club neighborhood that all the kids wanted to come to and play after school. But as much as I loved having a family, my marriage was just not right for me, or for my wife. Five years later, divorce was the right thing to do.

The process was horrible. I entered the darkest period of my life. During this same time, the daughter of an elderly patient had filed a complaint with the Texas Dental Board that I was doing more for her mother than what the daughter wanted. I immediately refunded her money, but the Texas Rangers still had to investigate the claim. I was in the midst of a suing my general contractor because the windows leaked in the large professional building I'd built. My office staff cruelly made me aware that the White Camellia Chapter of the Ku Klux Klan was active in Cleveland, and told me I should seek help from their Pentecostal Church. Everything that was dear to me was terribly torn apart. Eventually, I had to leave the town that I thought could never leave.

My divorce provided me with a push, though it wasn't a gentle one. In fact, it was more like a 2 x 4 between the eyes.

At first, I moved to a wealthy 'family-oriented' community north of Houston. My still-cloudy thinking told me this would be best for my daughter. But I was just miserable there: It was a sterile, lily-white, master planned community, and I felt more isolated than I had in Cleveland. I was flying back and forth to visit my daughter, and frantically doing everything I could for her. I fixed up her room and painted it pink before I even fixed up my own room. One day, a wonderful neighbor named Kay saw me running around at my usual breakneck pace. She said, "Randy, I see what you're doing. But Emily will be just fine as soon as Randy is just fine. Start figuring out what's best for you and the rest will fall into place." That turned out to be the best advice I ever received.

It was time to finally live my life with intention and purpose. I decided that I really needed to feel at home somewhere—and that somewhere was inside the Loop in Houston. I rented an apartment, then rented 900 square feet in a strip mall in a nice section of the city. I built that tiny strip mall space into a dental clinic and hung out my shingle again.

For about the next three years, there was very little time to focus much on me. My financial situation was pretty dire, and I was rebuilding my life and my practice from the ground up. I started working in a lock-up Alzheimer's facility just to have some steady income. I converted their beauty parlor into a MASH-style dental clinic and carried my instruments back and forth from my office.

At the same time, I was extremely committed to being a father to Emily. Her mother had moved her away to south of San Antonio; she was really trying to create any barriers she could for me to see my daughter. But I was going to be Emily's father, no matter what. That meant flying to San Antonio and bringing her back with me, then flying with her to San Antonio and flying back alone two to three times a month. There wasn't much money to do all that.

So I made yet another pivotal decision that it was time to focus what mattered the most to me: developing my practice in Houston, and being a father to my daughter. I sold my real estate back in Cleveland, breaking the last tie to the small town I'd left. Finally, I began living the life I was meant to live.

I can hear you saying to yourself right now, "All that stuff about deciding to do what's right sounds great. But it's the treatment *itself* that scares me. That's what stands in the way of my decision—it's the painful, frightening stuff."

By working together, we can find a way around the obstacles you're facing. I had a patient in my office the other day who can attest to that. He's been battling gum disease for years, and when we were in his treatment conference discussing some of the things I'd seen in his mouth, the gum disease topic came up. He told me. "I know it's back—my gums are bleeding again when I floss. In fact, I've pretty much quit flossing because the blood scares me. And I know you're going to tell me that I have to floss."

I said, "You didn't hear me say that. If I tell you to floss, is that going to make you do it?"

"No," he replied.

And I said, "Okay, then let's figure out some other way."

Battling gum disease is a battle against infection, and we can win it if we work together. If you had a splinter and it festered, you would get the splinter out and let your body heal. That's the basics of it. So my job is to do a deep cleaning—in effect, taking all of the splinters out from under your gums. If your gums are painful we'll make them numb so we can do a good job and not hurt you. But we'll physically clean out the infection we find and, afterwards, we'll fill up your toolkit with things you can do at home to heal yourself.

These tools will include some disinfecting mouthwashes. You may also take a prescription medication for two or three months, to reduce inflammation and help with the healing process. In addition, recommend you use an oral irrigator called a HydroFloss. It's a lot like a Waterpik, but it charges the ions in the liquid to kill bacteria. We offer nutritional supplements like probiotics to balance the good bacteria in your mouth and gut. You don't *have* to floss; it might make clearing up the infection more easily, but you don't have to do it.

That's step one—our Gums of Steel Program, which is pretty painless. Step two is to check you in a month or so to see how your gums have responded. Often, this two-step nonsurgical program is all you need to reverse the disease process. You'll just come back in regularly to get your teeth cleaned and stay on top of things. But if we're still seeing bleeding and inflammation, then we'll consider some laser therapy.

Lasers are another superior technology I use. They have all sorts of applications in industry, in medicine, and in dentistry. In periodontal therapy, they're used to kill the bacteria that hide in deep pockets of gum tissue. I've found laser therapy to be extremely effective at resolving gum disease once and for all. But in the most stubborn cases where gum disease persists, we don't give up hope. I work with an excellent periodontist, and have referred patients to this skilled gum disease specialist with incredible success.

As for treating dental decay and caries (the dentists' term for cavities), state of the-art-technologies make the process far friendlier than it has been for patients in the past. If you dread the process because you're imagining needle jabs, noisy drills, and gagging despite the little sucker apparatus that's stuck in your mouth, humor me for a minute and you'll see what I mean.

You've probably already caught on to the fact that I love changing people's perceptions about dentistry, and removing the obstacles to treatment that their past experiences have created. So let's imagine something different. Let's go get that cavity filled somewhere that doesn't smell like a dental office or look like one. Maybe it has some nice, soothing colors and a warm, welcoming feel about it. As part of your prep for that filling, let's do something really out of the box, like dip your hands in some hot paraffin wax and put some mittens over them. We'll put you in a chair, put some cushions up under your knees and behind your neck, wrap you up in a nice soft blanket, and take your shoes off and put some booties on your feet. We'll put some noise-cancelling headphones over your ears and put a little travel DVD up on the screen above your head.

Now let's rub some potent topical anesthetic on your gums, and instead of sticking you with a big needle, let's use a computer-aided device called 'the Wand' to administer more anesthetic into your gums. The Wand has a tiny tip that's going to deliver an anesthetic slowly, with gentle pressure, so you don't even know it's going in. But once it does, and you're really numb, we're going to put a little rubber drape over your tooth. It's going to keep all of the debris from falling into your mouth and down your throat—we won't put suckers down your throat to suck out all the goo.

As we work, you might feel a little vibration on that tooth, but there's no shrieking drill, and no creaking pressure as we put your filling in place. We're so gentle, and our technology is so advanced, that you're not going to have any of those sensations. We'll put in a tooth-colored filling, not a nasty-looking dark metal one. Then, we take the little drape off and guess what? We're finished.

At my office, you can literally rest easy.

HALITOSIS—IT'S MORE THAN BAD BREATH

With all of the high tech diagnostic tools at my disposal including digital x-rays, 3-D scans, EKGs, and DNA testing, one of the most reliable tools I have for diagnosing gum problems is my nose! Periodontal, or gum, disease is a bacterial gum infection. The bugs that cause it produce a pungent unique odor that is not from something you may have eaten like garlic, onions, coffee or alcohol.

The odor is caused by volatile sulphur compounds (VSCs) produced by bacteria that grow under the gums and in the pits and recesses of the tongue. Here are the basics on how to prevent that odor:

- **Brush your teeth and gums** at least twice a day.

- **Floss.** Or use a floss substitute like Hydrofloss or any other in between the teeth cleaner—that is where bacteria love to grow— places that are warm, dark, and moist.

- **Use a mouthwash.** But NOT the standard commercial ones. Most contain alcohol, which dries the mouth out and makes it worse after a short while. You need a mouthwash that kills or neutralizes the VSCs. Your dentist probably sells it. It contains chlorine dioxide, zinc ions, or sodium chlorite. One made with xylitol is even better! Xylitol is the next wave of innovative natural sweeteners made from plants that is actually good for you. (For more details on xylitol, see "Why Lube Is a Must.")

- **Scrape the crud off of your tongue.** It really is gross, and it stinks. Use a tongue scraper.

- **Suck on sugar-free mints.** Look for the natural sweetener xylitol in the ingredients.

While the steps above will keep your mouth fresh if you're in the lucky 10 percent of people who are free from periodontal disease, they aren't sufficient for the 90 percent of adults who have some form of gum disease (many of whom don't know it). This majority needs the help of a dentist or hygienist to get the bacteria and tartar cleaned off from under the gum line, and clear any infection from the gum tissue itself.

WHY LUBE IS A MUST

Why would a dentist be talking about lube? Because it turns out that in terms of oral health, lube is vitally important. The lube you need an abundance of: Saliva.

A lack of good saliva flow is the common denominator I see in patients who have the worst problems with gum disease, rampant cavities, and bad breath. Saliva is fluid that moisturizes the mouth, but it also does much more. It's made up of many enzymes, anti-bodies, and buffering agents. The enzymes and antibodies fight the harmful plaque, biofilms, bacteria, yeast, and fungus that can make their home on our teeth, tongue, and under the gum line. The buffer-ing agents neutralize the damaging acid pH of these nasty things.

People with an inadequate amount of saliva have a dry-mouth condi-tion called *xerostomia*. Xerostomia is damaging to both teeth and gums; plus, it's uncomfortable. It causes oral tissues such as the lips, tongue, and cheeks to stick together.

In researching an article that I wrote for MSN.com, I found an alarm-ing array of prescription drugs that turn off the saliva glands and sap saliva flow. High on the list: all antihistamines, almost all anti-depressants, and many high blood pressure medications, appetite suppressants, and narcotics. Other causes of dry mouth include smoking, excessive drinking, high amounts of caffeine, and use of mouthwashes with a high alcohol content. Radiation can also 'kill' sensitive saliva glands, so xerostomia often occurs in people who have had a cancer in the head and neck area that was treated with radiation.

Because Nature's lube is so critical to oral health, here's my advice: If you're taking medications that are sapping your saliva, talk with your physician to see if it is time to reduce the dosage or find something different. If you're suffering symptoms from self-inflicted causes (i.e., overuse of alcohol or caffeine), substitute for those harmful habits ones that do no harm. And if your xerostomia is caused by radia-tion therapy or something else out of your control, fight it! Sipping water frequently (and swishing it in your mouth before swallowing) is a good first step, as are over-the-counter artificial oral lubricants (like those made by Biotene and Spry). *(continued on next page...)*

But if your lube's running low, it's even more important than usual that your oral hygiene be meticulous, and that your regular dental cleanings include fluoride treatments. Your dentist should also check the pH of your saliva, and prescribe remineralizing agents such as MI paste, if necessary. Another best-kept secret: Using a natural sweetener called xylitol. It is plant derived and contains very few calories—and in the mouth, it balances pH, stimulates saliva, and fights bad bacteria. For xylitol that you can use just like sugar, check the health food section of better grocery stores. And ask your dentist to supply you with chewing gum, breath mints, and toothpastes made with xylitol. It tastes great, and is great for you!

WHICH TOOTHPASTE SHOULD I USE?

This is an incredibly common question I get from patients—and because good oral hygiene is a cornerstone of general dentistry, I wanted to address that question here. Once again, my answer may surprise you: You really don't need toothpaste at all to properly clean your teeth.

Toothpaste manufacturers use a not-so-secret formula for making their products. To describe it, I use the acronym **SOAP,** which stands for **Surfactants, Other thickeners, Abrasives, and Perfume**. None of those ingredients are considered 'active.' They just put on a show.

Surfactants are detergents like sodium laurel sulphate. It is used in many types of cleansers, especially shampoo and laundry detergent, and many people are sensitive to it. People that are sensitive to it will have breakouts around their waist where their clothing presses against the skin. They are shocked when I tell them that the skin around their mouth also breaks out with the sodium laurel sulfate that most toothpastes contain.

Other thickeners are gums, humectants, glycerin, and similar ingredients used to help make toothpaste bubble or foam. *(continued on next page...)*

Abrasives can be downright damaging to teeth. Many of the abrasives in 'whitening' toothpastes can scratch tooth enamel or the porcelain that is used for crowns and veneers. They're a lot like the Comet or Dutch cleanser everyone used to clean sinks and toilets when I was a kid; they were so abrasive they made things look clean, but destroyed the glaze on the porcelain so it had a dull finish.

Perfumes and sweeteners are added to commercial toothpastes to mask the yucky taste of the gums, surfactants, and humectants.

The only active ingredient that really does any good is **fluoride.** When added to toothpaste formulations, it helps prevents cavities by adding this important mineral back to tooth enamel. I do use toothpaste because it is convenient and tastes good and has fluoride in it. But the ones I use, Cloysis or Spry, don't contain sodium laurel sulphate.

I also occasionally make a homemade paste out of baking soda, salt, and hydrogen peroxide. That really helps kill bacteria and will actually whiten teeth without hurting the enamel or porcelain. My recipe is really pretty simple: Just put one or two teaspoons of baking soda in a small dish, sprinkle in a few grains of salt, and add enough hydrogen peroxide to make a thick slurry or paste.

I also tell patients that using the right toothBRUSH is far more important than using the 'right' toothpaste. These days all toothbrushes are made out of a nylon bristle. The only difference between and soft, medium, or hard bristle is the diameter of each little bristle. The hard bristle is thicker so it does not bend easily. The soft bristle is very narrow so it bends easily and feels soft. The smaller—and, thus, softer—the bristle, the better it is at getting the plaque and biofilms cleaned from the teeth. That is what is really important! The better brushes also have polished rounded edges on the bristle. Those cost more to make, so the brushes are priced a bit more. But they are worth the extra money.

CHAPTER 5

NeuroMuscular Dentistry: The Answer to Jaw Pain— and Much, Much More!

"I'm a mess!"

Those were Cindy's words—not mine. I heard them when she was forced to see me and undergo emergency dental surgery for a broken tooth in her 'smile zone'. I call the smile zone the teeth that show when you are talking and smiling, and in my office, a broken or missing tooth there is considered an emergency. The other thing we deem an emergency is severe pain. Cindy had both.

Cindy's hectic and stressful job left her little time for basic maintenance, much less self-improvement—and like many people in such a situation, her teeth bore testament. Besides the pain of the broken tooth, she was suffering from nearly debilitating facial muscle discomfort because of TMD—Temporo Mandibular Disorder. TMD is a malfunction or disharmony of the jaw joints, facial muscles, and bite. The muscle pain it causes can be extremely severe.

But perhaps the biggest pain Cindy endured was emotional pain. Like many people, she was terrified of going to the dentist. Little wonder that it took a broken tooth to get her to pay some badly needed attention to her smile and to her overall dental health.

Ultimately, all of Cindy's dental problems were corrected. I fitted her with an orthotic to get relief from the TMD pain, and then corrected her bite with Invisalign braces. The one thing I could not overcome, even with all of the great new technology I have to help suppress pain and discomfort, was her very real fear of seeing a dentist. We had to work on that together; it required her participation.

To get through her initial emotional and physical pain, Cindy had IV Sedation for her first emergency implant surgery. Then the LifeSmiles Experience, or 'the magic' happened. Cindy trusted me to be honest and direct with her, and to not hurt her. Once I gained her trust during her first appointment, she did not need sedation for anything else!

I see fear much like Cindy's in patients regularly. I understand it, and I approach it from the standpoint that I can help you overcome it by respecting that fear—and then demonstrating how I will simply not allow pain to be an obstacle for you. I won't allow it to prevent you from experiencing the satisfaction of overall well-being that fixing your dental problems will accomplish.

Cindy doesn't hesitate to pay a visit to LifeSmiles for her routine dental checkups now, and exudes a far different attitude than she had at our first encounter. As Cindy herself put it recently in a note to me:

> *Glad that I chose to come to you over two years ago when I was in bad shape. We've come a long, long way, haven't we? Everyone notices my smile now. Even better, the intense pain in my jaw and in my facial muscles is gone. Thanks, Dr. M, for all you've done to improve my quality of life. I actually look forward to come to the dentist's office now—it used to be something I absolutely dreaded.*

There's more to this transformation, though. Successfully facing down one fear arms us with new tools to face other fears and phobias. Cindy really did accomplish much more when she slayed that 'fear dragon'. She also quit the job that was such a major stress in her life and is truly a different woman today.

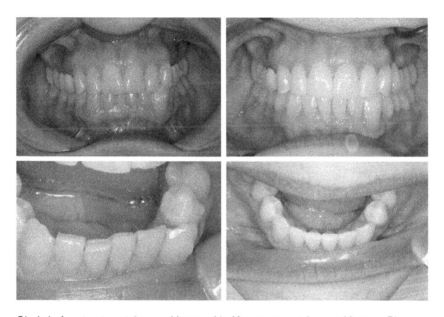

Cindy before treatment (top and bottom L); After treatment (top and bottom R)

To read more about Cindy's story and to discover how to give those pesky headaches and irritating jaw pain the knockout blow just visit **www.lifesmiles.us/jawpain**

I recently saw another patient who had a classic complaint. He told me, "For quite some time, I can make my jaw pop when I open it a certain way. The other day I had these crazy deadlines to meet for work that super stressed me out, and all of a sudden, I could not close my teeth together. The harder I tried to close them, the more it hurt." Though his symptoms were somewhat different than Cindy's, he too was suffering from a case of Temporomandibular Joint Dysfunction, or TMD.

The problem used to be called TMJ; short for TemporoMandibular Joint, or the jaw joint itself. It's the most complex joint in the human body, and is not a 'ball and socket' type joint. Remember the pictures in grade school how a snake can unhinge its jaw and swallow an entire egg or a rat? The human jaw joint (or joints, since there are two) has a similar action. When you open and close your mouth, it acts like a hinge.

Try this: Put your fingers just in front of your ear and feel for the joint. Now open wide like you're yawning or taking a bite of a Big Mac. You'll feel the joint actually unhinge and move forward over a hump. A very thin disc inside that joint works in harmony with many different muscles to make that happen smoothly. The popping sound my patient reported is the disc popping in and out between the bones. The pain and inability to put his teeth together is caused by a muscle spasm; it actually has nothing to do with the joint itself at all. That is why the name was changed from TMJ to TMD, to describe a dysfunction of the entire apparatus.

Most people can have 'jaw popping' for years and suffer no other obvious symptoms. The trouble occurs when you either wear a hole in the disc, or overstretch the muscles and ligaments that draw the disc back into place. Then, all of a sudden, you cannot close your teeth, or it is really difficult to chew. And it can hurt a lot! Ask me how I know.

A while back, I had a pain in my knee that was so bad I could barely walk across the room. I went to see my chiropractor, who diagnosed it as a muscle problem. He started working on 'stripping out' the muscles of my leg, using deep massage-type strokes to stretch out the muscle spasms. His treatment hurt like hell. I couldn't believe this level of pain was caused by muscles, and insisted that I probably needed surgery. So he did an MRI. It proved him right—the knee joint itself was perfectly okay. All of the pain was of muscle origin.

To treat TMD, I have developed innovative techniques in what we call neuromuscular dentistry. The goal of neuromuscular dentistry is to correct disharmony between the muscles of the face and the jaw joint by correcting your bite, or the way your teeth fit together. If your teeth don't fit together properly, your jaw joint and muscles can't work in true harmony. Most people adapt to the disharmony for a while, but it takes its toll over time. One day, the body can't take it anymore and things flare up. It shows up several ways—in addition to the problems I've already described, you can suffer muscle tension headaches, ringing in the ears, facial fatigue upon wakening (from grinding your teeth through the night), and worn-down, as well as chipped, teeth.

To get the information needed to re-establish harmony, we use a computer to take EMGs (electromyography readings that measure muscle activity of the face, much like an EKG measures the heart). We also use a technology called TekScan that involves biting down on a paper-thin plastic circuit board. This yields precise measurements of how the teeth bite together, and is much more precise than the old-fashioned method of biting down on carbon paper.

We typically use a combination of several approaches to correct a bad bite. Those might include orthodontics to move the teeth into a better position, spot-grinding teeth that are out of place and causing muscle imbalances, making an orthotic that's much like some people put in their shoe to level their hips, or putting new biting surfaces on the teeth to make them fit in harmony with the joint and muscles.

My expertise in neuromuscular dentistry allows me to use techniques even in patients who don't have TMD. In fact, I employ principles when I do implants, dentures, even the dental facelifts described in several cases in this book. Whenever I work on patients, ensuring the proper balance between the teeth, jaw, and muscles is a key concern. My attention to this balance yields a better-looking, better-feeling, and all-around sounder and healthier result.

For more information on neuromuscular dentistry and the difference it can make for you, check out the Special Report on my website at www.lifesmiles.us/TMD

CHAPTER 6

Still Hate the Thought of Going to the Dentist? Rethink What You're Really Worth

I am extremely grateful that the majority of my patients have above average intelligence—however, that sometimes actually makes them 'bad patients.' It may shock you to hear me use that term, but let me define what I mean by this: I have found that, sometimes, a high IQ conflicts with what people psychologically feel they deserve for themselves. Sometimes, a high IQ teaches them hard lessons about themselves. To illustrate what I mean, let me tell you about one of my patients.

Sam had the means to get anything he needed or wanted in life, but he had neglected his teeth for nearly 20 years. His personal lesson hit home on the day he realized that the same logic he applied to keeping his beautiful black Mercedes in top running condition should also apply to his own running condition.

It took a warning from his doctor for Sam to come and see me. When we discussed the dental work he needed, he questioned the cost— or, more accurately, he questioned his own hesitation to make the investment in himself. "I've got this really great-looking car, but frankly, my own appearance is really kind of embarrassing," he admitted. "Why is it that I won't even bat an eye when the dealership tells me it'll cost over

$2,500 for a minor repair on my car—and yet I'm struggling to justify paying money to take care of my dental problems?"

"Which will ultimately be more important in your life?" I asked Sam. "Your Mercedes, or your teeth?"

It comes down to the value we place on ourselves, based on the confidence we have in ourselves. Our smiles convey our personal confidence, perhaps more than any other outward action we can make. So if we don't smile, our self-confidence dims. Then the process feeds on itself. The more we fail to smile, the more our confidence shrinks. Over time, even the most intelligent among us can come to undervalue ourselves so much that we come to believe it's not worth investing in our smiles—even though that's the very thing we should do.

The important point is that even these 'bad patients'—those highly intelligent people I see with misplaced perceptions—can easily be shown that investing in their own teeth ultimately shows a higher return. Sam found that out. He made the investment and had his dental work completed. As an attorney for a large energy company, he now uses his smile every day—and he tells me it was the best money he ever spent.

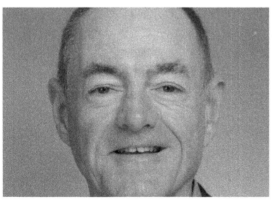 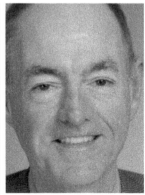

Sam before treatment (L); After treatment (R)

To read more about Sam's story and to discover the path to realizing a higher self-worth visit **www.lifesmiles.us/worth**

THE ROAD NOT TAKEN

Growing up, I wasn't the 'bad kid' in my family, but even as a 'good kid,' I always felt different. Deep inside, I knew I wanted something more than a blue-collar life, but I didn't really see my own potential. I didn't see myself as a wise investment—yet.

Then one summer when I was a teen, I went to church camp for a week. I'd always loved going to church. Everything was good there—it was good to be good, and good to be honest. I believe that going to church grounded me in goodness. It also exposed me to seeing people who lived the kind of life that life was supposed to be about.

At church camp, I met a Reverend W.C. Hall, Jr. I had never known anyone like him. He was so smart! He genuinely cared about me, what I thought about things, and what my feelings were. He asked me about my plans to go to college (I had none at the time). He had a white German Shepherd named Sampson that was trained better than any circus act I had ever seen.

W.C. had a history of helping disadvantaged kids, and he took me under his wing. He showed me a world I didn't know existed—exposed me to theater and music and nice clothes and going places; taught me how to order in a restaurant and how to enjoy a glass of wine. I still remember the first I ever tasted—a rosé from Portugal called Mateus, served in an oval green bottle.

Through W.C., I learned that such things weren't sinful or wasteful. It was entirely okay to enjoy what people call 'the finer things in life'—and to enjoy life itself. He accepted my intelligence and love for learning; in fact, he valued it. He informed me that it was time for me to take college entrance exams, visit, and apply to colleges. He picked me up and took me to tour my first college campus. I was in awe—it was yet another world I had never known about.

W.C. was the most amazing person this young geek had ever met. He was intelligent, educated, cultured, and greatly respected by his church members. In fact, he was a big reason that I declared my intention to become a Methodist minister. While that path didn't pan out, I give W.C. enormous credit for changing the course of my life. His investment in me taught me that I was worth it. Because of him, I went from being a common worker to becoming the successful dentist I am today.

Speaking of 'bad patients'—and by 'bad,' I continue to mean those who don't see themselves as a wise investment—brings me to the story of my own mother. She suffered with this misplaced perception so much! As you may recall, I grew up as the second oldest of five children in a lower-middle-class family. Mom had her hands full raising that many kids on a small budget. Dental care for everyone was pretty far down on the list—with her being at the bottom of that list. Thankfully, she kept her teeth very clean. Still, she lost a number of them along the way.

Now, dentists' mothers get very good deals on dental work from their kids, and I've been my mom's dentist for more than 25 years now. But for the majority of those years, all she ever wanted was patchwork dentistry. Granted, she is exquisitely sensitive to pain, and her son is exquisitely sensitive to her squirming. But those weren't the driving forces behind her dental decisions. Like Sam and so many other people, she could not convince herself that having a beautiful smile was truly something she deserved to have. That's a struggle for people—a realization they still find difficult, even when their dental work is something they can easily afford.

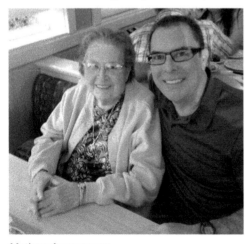
Mother after veneers

The good thing about the only type of 'bad patient' I've ever come across is that it's never too late to see the light. Even my stubborn mother did. At 81 years of age, my mother finally reached the point that she was ready to give herself permission to have her mouth fixed the way she really wanted. I was able to remove a bad tooth, place a number of dental implants, and give her the smile her own son knew she always deserved. She was extremely comfortable through the whole thing, as was I! And IV sedation was the reason.

There are a lot of reasons that even people who want to invest in themselves are apprehensive about going to the dentist. Fear of being lectured, fear of needles, even a history of negative, painful dental experiences as a child are just a few. The ability of the kind of sedation dentistry I do to overcome such apprehension is why I'm so proud to offer it.

You may know people who take their dogs and cats into the vet to have their teeth cleaned—in fact, you may be an animal lover who's had your own pet's dental work done. Often, the pet is sedated for the procedure. You spend a few hundred dollars extra for the sedation, and typically, you don't do it to make the vet's job easier. You do it because you know going to the vet stresses out your pet, and you want to save them that stress. Why not give yourself the same break and consider sedation dentistry for yourself?

Sedation dentistry is incredibly effective, but first, let me forewarn you: You've undoubtedly heard dentists advertising it on the radio, or have seen it promoted on the Internet or in the phone book. Most of these advertisements are for conscious sedation; some even use the terms 'sleep' to mislead people into believing that they will be asleep during their dental appointment. The majority of dentists who advertise such services use a combination of nitrous oxide gas and pills—relaxation produced by pills. These pills work for some people, but not all. Often, they are not adequate for those who have true anxiety over dental procedures. Plus, you really do not know their effects until almost an hour after you take them. If those effects aren't adequate, you are just out of luck. You either cancel the work or the dentist does it anyway.

I am one of the very few prestigious dentists licensed and trained to administer sedation both with pills and deeper IV sedation. The Texas Dental Board only awards licensing to those who have undergone extensive rigorous training, amassed clinical experience, and provided proof of their skills in these techniques. This means the sedation dentistry I offer is much more advanced than what most dentists do. Through the sedation I use, you have little or no memory of having any dental work done, and experience minimal if any discomfort or pain.

I go one step further. I also offer the option of taking a prescription medication an hour before your appointment so you will be relaxed by the time you arrive at my office. (Since you will be sedated, you will need someone to drive you to and from the appointment.) You will be seated in a chair and made comfortable with things like a warm blanket, booties on your feet, memory foam pillows, even sunglasses to protect you from the bright lights we use to do your dental work.

We'll then use an IV to administer a sedative directly into your bloodstream. Intravenous sedation is safer and more predictable than is oral sedation alone. Not only can the level of sedation be controlled much more accurately, but the drugs can also be reversed if necessary. Furthermore, your vital signs are monitored just as they would be in a hospital setting, using telemetry that measures your EKG, pulse, heart rate, oxygen level, and breathing rate.

Sedation dentistry can be used in a wide variety of situations. It's ideal for patients who've had bad dental experiences in the past, those who have trouble getting numb, those who fear needles, and/or those who are anxious or embarrassed about their teeth. It's also adaptable to any kind of dental work. Patients who have limited time can use it to have a lot of their dental work done in a single session, rather than a series of appointments. Others will use it for more simple procedures, such as regular cleanings.

To learn more about the many applications of sedation dentistry, and what LifeSmiles' advanced techniques can do for you, refer to my Special Report at www.lifesmiles.us/gotosleep

When Teeth Aren't Lasting as Long as You Hoped: Restoring Your Smile, Rebuilding Your Life

Sue had spent her life taking excellent care of her husband and four children, but for 52 years had only had 'patchwork' dentistry done for herself. When her front tooth broke off, she was embarrassed for anyone to see her. Her husband did an Internet search for the best implant dentist, found my website and called my office.

Even though Sue was in no pain, we saw her right away, since I consider a lost front tooth to be a dental emergency. We did a thorough examination; then, Sue, her husband, and I had a heart-to-heart talk. The 3-D digital x-ray had revealed a number of serious dental problems, and Sue herself confided to me that she was pretty anxious about having dental work done. Together, we reached a decision: We would remove her broken-down teeth, place the latest generation of technologically advanced dental implants, and attach new teeth to the implants all in the same day.

Then the 'magic' started to unfold. Digital photos were matched to the 3-D x-rays, models made and new teeth were sculpted even before her implants were placed. This is different from the way most dentists

*proceed—they place the implants first, and then decide where the new
teeth go. Often, this results in the new teeth not being in the perfect place
to create a beautiful smile. I know that optimally placed teeth dictate
where the implants should be placed, so I work in that order.*

*On the day her implants were placed, Sue was made extremely com-
fortable with IV Sedation. Her damaged teeth were removed and the
dental implants were inserted using computer-guided imagery; no large
surgical incisions had to be made. The new teeth (which had already
been carefully designed) were then attached to the implants. Within a few
hours, Sue walked to the car with her new smile. Afterward, she reported
taking only one pain pill.*

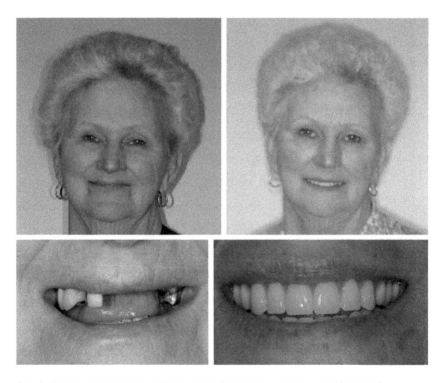

Sue before treatment (top and bottom L); After treatment (top and bottom R)

To read more about Sue's story and to discover how restoring your smile
can build a better life, visit **www.lifesmiles.us/restore**

Even though preserving your natural teeth is a top priority for me, sometimes teeth just can't be saved. Still, that doesn't constitute failure or disaster for you, *or* for me. In reality, restoring lost teeth is a process of rebuilding. And I'm living proof that in rebuilding, we can realize our dreams.

I started from ground zero in my Houston practice. I didn't buy into someone else's practice or look for an associate because I had made a pledge to myself: I would make this new practice the true embodiment of ideal dentistry. I would make my own decisions about the services I offered, the people I hired, and the patients I chose to treat. I was focused on living my mission in life: To build up people and create beautiful things.

And my practice blossomed. I was finally able to be the highly advanced dentist that I had trained to be. I had been frustrated back in that small town where few people had an appreciation for the best dentistry that could be done. Most were satisfied with mediocre dentistry. I wanted to perform the best dentistry, and be the best dentist possible, so my patients could have the very best.

It did not take long for my reputation as an outstanding and caring dentist to spread. I had to move to a larger building. I closed my eyes and envisioned what my ideal dental office would look like. That vision had hardwood floors, a fireplace, columns, nice land-scaping, a tastefully designed space, and did not smell like a dental office. With this vision in mind, I drove around my favorite part of town and spotted a rundown building for sale. It was much more expensive than what I thought I could afford, but the minute I walked in it clicked. This was the place I had seen in my vision. It took a year to transform the 1930s, two-story duplex home into one of the most unique dental offices in the country. During the process, my decorator, Tony Huffman, suggested I live in the upstairs space.

I had planned to rent out that space but said to myself, "Why not?" I'm glad I made that decision; it's a wonderful place to live. And for patients, it's a wonderful place to visit. The look out over tropically landscaped pool as they receive the most advanced dental services possible. With the use of 3-D digital x-ray CT scans, 3-D images instead of gooey impressions, CAD/CAM designs, EMGs, computer bite analysis, and state-of-the-art techniques in cosmetic dentistry and dental implant surgery, my patients get outstanding results that look good, feel good, and last a long time.

They also get the benefit of a dentist who cares, and who demonstrates his dedication by continuing to learn the latest advancements in the field. I am the only dentist in the world with a Masters honor from both the American Academy of General Dentistry *and* The American Dental Implant Association. In addition, I am one of the very few general dentists with these credentials who is certified and licensed to give my patients IV Sedation. This assures them the most comfortable experience possible for any procedure, not just surgery.

As for myself, yes, I'm still learning. And I always will be—not only about dentistry, but also about myself. For me, there is a blurry line between what some people would call work and what I call play. But I've achieved a sense of peace about the balance of work and play, and love and worship, in my life. I have come to conclude that the center point of balance is pinned down at different places for different people, and my center point is right for me. Life is good, and I am grateful.

I do believe our Creator had a pretty clever design. We get two sets of teeth to start with. You get to totally screw things up until the age of 6 years, when that first set begins to get lost. Then you're issued a 'get out of jail free' card and the clock starts ticking on the second set. The dilemma is, when will that clock run out?

Technically, a full house of permanent teeth numbers 32. However, most people have the wisdom teeth removed and some people are born without all four wisdom teeth. Therefore, I do not include wisdom teeth in my count of what is considered a 'full set.' So, you get one last free pass. A full set is considered 28 teeth.

Of the 315 million Americans currently living, 178 million are missing at least one tooth (http://www.gotoapro.org/news/facts--figures/). The interesting thing is that once a person loses one tooth and doesn't have it replaced, the odds of entering the next category—of missing two or more teeth—skyrockets. In effect, losing one tooth and not replacing it can put you on a slippery slope to more rapid tooth loss.

Tooth Replacement Options: The Basics

There are several different methods to replace missing teeth, all of which I offer to my patients. The least-expensive option is to fit you with a "flipper," a removable partial denture that can be used to replace one to four missing teeth. A flipper is made of rigid plastic, and snaps onto adjacent teeth. It usually covers part of your palate, sort of like the orthodontic retainer you might have had as a kid. Flippers aren't my favorite option. They're a bit awkward to wear, and often require denture adhesive to hold them in place. Their rigid plastic is somewhat porous, so over time it can develop a smell. Plus, it isn't particularly durable, so flippers can break easily. Still, they have their advantages. You can take them easily out to clean them, and when cost is a big concern, they're literally smile-savers.

Bridges are another replacement method. These are partial dentures that 'dock,' if you will, onto the teeth on either side of the gap created by your missing tooth (or teeth). To achieve this docking, we drill down those adjacent teeth, fit them with crowns, and anchor the bridge onto them. Bridges can be made and 'docked,' crowns included, pretty quickly. You're all said and done in a matter of two or three weeks. Their disadvantage is that we have to cut down the two adjacent teeth of the space made by the missing tooth. These adjacent teeth may be perfectly good healthy teeth. If you have a failure (meaning a cavity,) on one of those caps, the entire apparatus fails. You lose the whole bridge and have to have a new one remade, which means you have to grind down another tooth to cap it. And if that cap fails, you're into somewhat of a domino effect.

On the plus side, bridges are less bulky and more durable than flippers. And they won't fall out and embarrass you, as flippers sometimes can. On the minus side, they're more difficult to clean. But all in all, bridges have served many people well for many years, so they're still a good option.

Implants—The Gold Standard

Both bridges and flippers have a somewhat limited lifespan of five to 20 years, which is a big reason why implants are far superior. Properly made and placed, the implants of today can last many more years than that. But there's a caveat: Even these state-of-the-art replacements require maintenance.

I've said it several times already: I'm a very honest person, and as your dentist, I'll always be honest with you. Don't let any dentist tell you anything he or she does to your teeth will last a lifetime. Do you remember when people would go to the beauty salon and get a 'permanent' for their hair? That hairdo lasted longer than a roller-set, but it certainly wasn't permanent. Some dentists use the term 'permanent' in a similar manner. They'll tell you the thing they want you to do is a 'permanent solution.' I'm here to tell you: I haven't seen any tooth replacement or restoration that can truly be expected to last a lifetime. However, dental implants do have a huge advantage in terms of longevity. And the ones I do have a number of other advantages, as well.

Implants come in two parts. Think of a dental implant as a titanium replacement of the *root* of a tooth in the jawbone. Because implants are anchored into the bone like the roots of your teeth, they act like natural teeth and preserve and strengthen the underlying bone. There is no need to drill down healthy teeth, and there are no plates to affect comfort and fit. Because the implant is like a root, you then can have a variety of options of what you attach to that root. It could be a single tooth, it could be used to lock down a loose denture, or you can place multiple implants to replace all of the teeth.

The typical way to place implants is to use a scalpel to make an incision in the gums, peel the gums away from the bone, and perform an osteotomy. That's the technical term for making a hole in the bone, and it's usually done free-hand. The implant is placed into the osteotomy, and the gums are sewn back into place. As the osteotomy heals, the implant is anchored into the bone. Once I've established the anchor is firm enough, I attach your new artificial tooth to the implant.

Depending on a patient's situation, I do perform such 'typical' implant surgeries. But in some cases, the ones I do are far more advanced. I am able to do them much like endoscopic surgery. Most of the time, an incision and stitches are no longer needed. This means there is very little discomfort and no bleeding.

The implants I do are computer-guided, and performed with the use of a cone-beam CT scan machine. This machine is actually just like the ones used to take CT scans of the heart and brain. In dentistry, we use it to get a 3-D image of the jaws. Then, on the computer monitor, we can take that image and spin it just like a 3-D Rubik's Cube. We can create a computer animation that places the implants on the monitor exactly where they need to go.

From this computer animation, we use a kind of 3-D printer to create a surgical guide. The guide will actually fit into the mouth so I can use it during implant surgery. It allows me to place the implants in the jawbone with great precision; I don't even have to cut the gums open. I simply punch a hole that's so tiny I don't even need to sew it up.

Computer-guided implants are a major leap forward in implant surgery, as are the way that implants themselves are now made. Over the years, they've gotten much smaller, and their surface is 'bio-attractive.' They attract the bone and the blood vessels to rapidly attach to them. Combined, these implant improvements translate to huge advantages for the patient in terms of time, pain, and swelling. You'll experience much less of those than you would have in the past. I tell my computer-guided implant patients they can expect little to no swelling or pain, and can return to normal eating the next day for single implants.

As far as the time from start to finish, in the past you would have the implant surgery, then wait almost six months to attach the teeth to it. Now, with modern implants and the techniques I use to place them, that process can take as little as eight weeks.

I'm the first to admit that there are exceptions; to get the results you deserve, the process cannot be rushed. Putting in an implant and the restoration that's placed on top of it is one of the most challenging procedures a dentist can do. I have to take into account how much bone you have in your jaw to anchor the implant; if there's not enough, you may need a bone graft before we can proceed. When I perform your implant surgery, I'll take every possible step to ensure healthy healing and successful 'anchoring' of the implant into the bone (including the use of tiny healing collars and Platelet Rich Plasma, a state-of the art substance derived from your own blood that plumps tissue to fill gaps between the implant and bone). Still, everyone heals at a different rate, and my honest nature won't allow me to promise you those superfast eight-week results in every case. What I can promise is that I'll discuss all details of your unique situation up front, and will stay with you along the way to make sure you're healing is progressing optimally.

I'll also put a lot of effort and skill into making your implants look good. In the early days of implants, they were considered successful if they just hung onto the bone. They weren't graded on how good they looked—dentists just did the happy dance if the bone healed well around them and they stayed firmly in place. Nowadays, that's just not enough. Your implant has to appeal to the eye and you need to be 100 percent satisfied with what your smile looks like. You can't just be satisfied that you've got a metal titanium implant that's hanging into the bone. Again, I can accomplish the excellence you deserve by designing your implants with the aid of CAD/CAM.

Dentures—They've Come a Long Way Since Grandma's Day

As superior and long-lasting as implants are, I realize that many people who need all or most of their teeth replaced can't reasonably afford a full set of implants. About 35 million Americans have no natural teeth left at all, and the majority of those folks wear dentures (http://www.gotoapro.org/news/facts--figures/).

Dentures can be a source of embarrassment; often, people who have them feel that they're looked down upon because they wear 'fake teeth.' The fact that I can help such people overcome those feelings, and introduce them to a better quality of life, makes denture-wearers some of my favorite patients.

I believe denture-wearers deserve the same fine care and respect as someone with perfect natural teeth. Unfortunately, most younger dentists receive little training in making and fitting dentures; as a result, they do not like making them. The consequence: I've seen far too many patients who've been handed a series of ill-fitting dentures made by several different dentists. These patients are desperate to find a dentist who understands them, and can help them. Thanks to my training and some exciting new technology, I'm proud to say I can do both.

I use a breakthrough technique called AvaDent to make dentures. 'Ava' means birth, 'Dent' means teeth—and AvaDent means the rebirth of your smile. It takes digital records of your jaws, face, and bite, and then creates a highly customized virtual denture right on the computer. Then, the denture is milled out of a solid block, yielding a result that is stronger than conventional acrylic dentures.

No dentures have ever looked and felt as real as those that AvaDent produces. It even matches the ridges in your palate and the texture of your gums to the parts of your denture that cover those areas. Unlike traditional dentures, AvaDents aren't made of porous material. This means they do not shrink, so you get a great, long-lasting fit. It also means they're more bacteria resistant, and don't develop the odor that gives conventional denture-wearers horrible breath. And while typical dentures take five appointments to make, AvaDent only requires two: One to make the records, the other to give you the final result. Those records, by the way, are all digital and kept on file. This means that if you lose or break your denture, a new one can be reproduced with the push of a button! I must admit, I also like the fact that AvaDent dentures are American made.

'ALL ON FOUR' SOUNDS FAST

The advertising sounds like a dream come true. A dentist is promising you the moon, telling you that by having dental implants done you can go from having ugly, miserable teeth to sporting a big beautiful smile in one day.

Remember that saying, "If it sounds too good to be true, it probably is"? Watch out!

Let me put it in plain English: These dentists invariably belong to high-advertising centers that employ a one-size-fits-all mentality to deliver a service known as 'all on four.' This means they treat all their patients the same—no matter how many teeth you have, even if many are in good condition, they take all of the teeth out to create a blank canvas. Then four implants are placed at whatever cock-eyed angle to reach into the jawbone to some degree. An acrylic denture is attached to those four implants, meaning all those teeth are anchored on four. The surgery itself may be done in one day, but the process involves a number of appointments leading up to that. Plus, the cost is typically $25,000 to $45,000 per upper or lower jaw, for a total of $50,000 to $95,000 (sometimes more).

Let's apply a little common sense to the math. Your Creator started you out with 14 teeth per arch (meaning 14 on top, and 14 on bottom) that can last a pretty long time. Now you are going to have four titanium implant screws do the work of 14. If you lose one natural tooth, it is not a disaster. But if you lose one of these four implants, it is beyond a disaster—it is a catastrophe! There is nowhere to go from there.

There is a better way to go. I listen to what the patient wants before I tell them what I can do. Most people want a nice smile, freedom of pain, and the minimum amount of dentistry done to achieve those goals. So sometimes, we leave teeth that are good and save money by not having to replace them. Sometimes, we do just the top arch of teeth first, or just the teeth that are in the smile zone first. Then we give options of doing the back teeth later, if that fits the budget better. *(continued on next page...)*

Everything starts with an accurate diagnosis and assessment of what your current conditions are, what your short and long term goals for your teeth and smiles are, and what fits your budget. Many times all of the teeth do not have to be taken out, which saves you both money and future problems.

In cases where it really is best to remove all of the teeth, I typically place two to four times as many implants. When possible, you'll have 'all on' 6, 8, or 10 implants instead of 'all on four.' This preserves the jaw bone (since the bone that grows around the implants doesn't shrink the way that bone can when dentures are just sitting on top of them). It also gives you a backup system—if one or more of your implants ever develops a problem, you'll have more to provide your dentures with support. Often, rather than using a one-piece denture, we can take a modular approach, placing individual teeth or bridges supported by implants. As repairs or replacements are needed in the future, you have lots of options left open.

And here's the real kicker: Typically, I can do the entire job for you at the same or lower cost than that big center advertised. The computer-guided implant surgery I do is actually quite cost-effective compared to conventional implant surgery. It offers better value, because the bridges and dentures I use can be made of milled zirconium, which lasts a lot longer than conventional acrylic (and doesn't develop a smell!). I also do not have the high overhead costs of expensive TV ads, and don't have to pay into a big corporate structure. I can pass those savings along to you. I can treat you as an individual, working with you to find the solution that's best for you. Dentistry is never a one-size-fits-all proposition. Never, ever settle for anything less than a highly personalized plan.

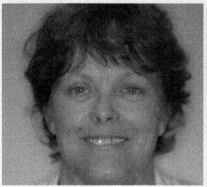 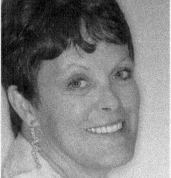

Sue before treatment (L); After treatment (R)

CHAPTER EIGHT

Cosmetic Dentistry: Because Confidence Counts

Carol called the office and said that she wanted six porcelain veneers on her upper front teeth. Could she have that?

The answer: Of course she could!

We did not know it at the time, but my office was the sixth dental office that Carol had called. We did not know she had already been to five other dentists and made the same simple question. And we did not know that each of those five previous dentists had, upon examining Carol, refused her request.

Those dentists dogmatically explained to Carol that she had back teeth with excessive abscesses, and those should be her immediate concern. Her priority, they told her, shouldn't be the cosmetic beautification of her six front teeth.

But Carol didn't want the badly abscessed back teeth repaired first. She wanted six front porcelain veneers. So, with increasing amounts of frustration, she paid a series of five consultation fees, leaving each time without those six porcelain veneers on her upper front teeth.

When Carol arrived for her appointment and I saw the terrible condition of the rest of her teeth, I too told her that, by law, I needed to inform her of her other more pressing health issues. However, I then did something that five other dentists simply refused to do: I told Carol that if there were reasons why she truly felt she needed to have the veneers done before taking care of her other serious dental issues, that was her choice to make. We would honor that choice.

Carol was startled. "You will do it? Just my front teeth, right?"

I assured her that the answer was a simple, "Yes."

She then pulled out a photograph and said, "This is what I want them to look like, and I need it done rather quickly."

I won't deny that I would have preferred to have Carol ask us to resolve her other dental problems first—but there was no reason to refuse her request, no matter how odd it seemed. So the front teeth were cleaned and prepared to receive the six very white porcelain veneers. The underlying teeth were so badly broken down it was necessary to cover them with temporary acrylic veneers while the porcelain was being made in the lab. Even these temporary veneers looked very nice.

A few weeks later, it was time to bond the porcelain veneers onto her teeth. This was a challenge, because all of the rest of the teeth were in such poor condition, but the appointment went smoothly and did not take long. Soon, it was time to freshen up Carol's face with a warm, scented towel, sit her up in the dental chair, and let her see her new look in a large hand mirror.

It's always exciting for my team to witness the transformation from something that looks 'not so pretty' to something that looks downright beautiful—yet at the same time looks anything but artificial. We watched as Carol took a deep breath, raised the mirror to look at herself, and started crying. It's not uncommon for both men and women to get emotional at the transformation they see, but Carol did not just cry. She wept. Then she sobbed uncontrollably.

My dental team and I feared the worst. Did she absolutely hate what she saw? When she finally was able to control herself, I gingerly asked, "Carol, what's wrong with them?"

"Absolutely nothing," Carol said. "They are beautiful and exactly what I want."

With that statement, she pulled off her wig to reveal little sprigs of thin hair. And only then did she finally tell me why those six veneers were so damned important to her.

"The rest of my teeth don't matter," Carol explained. "Eight months ago, I was told that I had only six months to live because of cancer. I'm already living on borrowed time. But you see, I used to secretly work as a double for one of our first ladies. Next week, I am to be honored at a dinner at the White House for that work." She smiled and her new beautiful front teeth gleamed. "There will be lots of photographers and I will have my picture taken. It's bad enough that I have no hair. I at least wanted a nice smile."

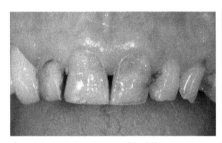 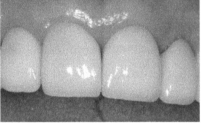

Carol before treatment (L); After treatment (R)

Carol's story is very important to me because it illustrates what I strongly believe: Assumptions and judgment about the priorities of our patients have no place in my office. It is very dangerous to presume that I know why people make the decisions they do. You never know what circumstances they may have in their life. Our job, and our first responsibility to you, is to help you restore your confidence according to the priorities you give us.

To read more about Carol's story and to discover the power of a confident smile visit **www.lifesmiles.us/confidence**

The confidence that Carol gained from the cosmetic procedures we performed was especially meaningful to her, given the state of her mouth and her health. But even people who have generally healthy teeth and gums can benefit from the boost in confidence that state-of-the-art cosmetic dentistry provides. A lot of research has been done to prove your smile is one of the first things people look at. You have about 10 seconds to make that first impression, and when cosmetic procedures help people feel great about the look of their smiles, I've literally seen their lives take off.

Whiter Teeth Through Bleaching

Today, it is considered good grooming to have healthy, clean teeth; dingy or yellowed teeth are simply not acceptable. I won't get into whether I consider it right or wrong, but the fact is that most people make judgments of others based on their personal appearance, and a white smile is considered more attractive. A recent *Wall Street Journal* survey proved that all other things being equal, attractive people make more money and have an easier time attracting someone than do less-attractive people.

The first question to answer if you want your teeth whiter is how white do you want them? This is a matter of personal preference. Some patients want a little freshening-up, while others want blindingly white—like, I need to put my sunglasses on because your teeth are glowing!

You can get a whitening effect from some of the over-the-counter products on the market. Just don't buy some of the infomercial products and other cheap stuff that may have ingredients like citric acid. The acid whitens teeth by making them frosty, like etched glass. That is bad for tooth enamel. The major brands of whitening systems are kinder to enamel. They cost around $100, and at best will leave teeth mildly whiter. The reason: Their real whitening ingredient is oxygen. It is bound up in various concentrations of either hydrogen peroxide or carbamide peroxide, and releases when applied to the teeth. These are highly unstable chemicals that release the oxygen very easily and quickly. The oxygen is destroyed by water, saliva, and heat.

Therein lays the problem. These products get manufactured and sent to a HOT warehouse. Then they get shipped and sit in the HOT delivery truck. Then they might sit in your car in the Texas heat until you get home. By that time, most of the effectiveness is lost due to exposure to heat. Also, the strips or do-it-yourself trays do not seal at the gum line, so the material oozes out or lets saliva get into the tray. After 10 minutes in the mouth under those conditions, you may as well take it out of your mouth and throw it away. It's done.

Tray-based bleaching systems offered by dentists give better whitening results. We use professional-strength bleach and make custom-fitted trays that keep saliva out. (Because the bleach is strong, we also protect the cheek and gums from exposure to it.) Sometimes, a powerful light is applied to release the oxygen faster. The cost will be $350–$750.

A few dentists that are serious about whitening—myself included—offer a system known as Kor bleaching to their patients. It is called deep bleaching because its oxygen is absorbed more deeply into the tooth. This means it can erase deeper stains. The product is refrigerated every step of the way, from manufacturer to dentist to patient. The custom-made trays that are proprietary for this system have a special seal at the gum line to keep saliva out. The Kor system guarantees results—that's huge, since guarantees for whitening have been unheard of until now. The cost of Kor ranges from about $850–$1,500, depending on the number of visits required.

Whiter Teeth Through Veneers

Veneers are basically thin porcelain covers for your teeth. They certainly can give teeth a whiter appearance, since they cover your natural stained or dingy surface. But they can also be used to correct problems such as ridges, pitting or ragged, uneven edges on teeth. They can also be used to correct the bite.

Lumineers is a well-marketed brand of porcelain veneers, developed by a dental laboratory in California. I wish their product were as good as their marketing.

Lumineers are promoted as the way to a low-cost beautiful smile with no drills and no shots. Once again, if it sounds too good to be true, it probably is. The system involves creating a porcelain shell that is bonded over teeth, cavities, old fillings, and crooked teeth. But Lumineers are much like Lee Press On Nails. While they're fine for some people, they're not customizable. They all look extremely white and opaque. Plus, they're thicker than natural teeth, so they can create a surface up against the gum that sets the stage for bacteria to breed. I have seen a number of patients who've had Lumineers done, and I've had the unfortunate task of telling them they now have gingivitis (or worse) and will need to have their teeth redone with a better-designed porcelain veneer.

This raises an important point: When done properly, cosmetic dentistry not only looks good, it is good *for* your teeth. The dentist who performs your cosmetic work should have credentials that include special training in that work. Those credentials should come from respected institutions, not just a weekend seminar.

I find that my patients are typically more discriminating. When they seek out a smile enhancement, they want it to be beautiful and natural and fool the eye that anything has been done. The dentistry I perform is part science, part art. Giving you the best results involves a great deal of design work. With veneers, I could line them up like little soldiers if I wanted to—they'd look like perfect little Chicklets, but they wouldn't look real. To fool the eye in the most aesthetically pleasing way, I use customized porcelain veneers, designing them and applying them with meticulous attention to all the details.

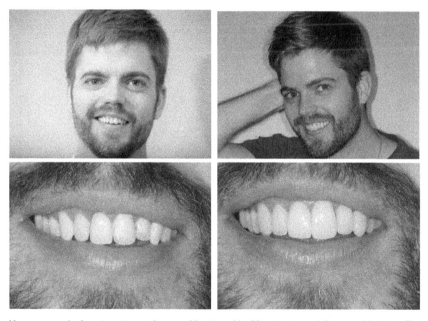

Young man before treatment (top and bottom L); After treatment (top and bottom R)

This attention includes cleaning out any cavities and old fillings that might be on the teeth before we even start, and then designing your smile according to the Old Master's technique of Golden Proportions. For a beautiful smile, proper shape of each individual tooth is just as important as the color of the teeth, if not more so. If the teeth are not straight, we will either move the teeth with orthodontics or braces, or polish them down to first get them in alignment.

Then, we will work with an exceptionally talented and well-trained dental lab that understands the artistic side of cosmetic dentistry. The veneers they make for my patients are thinner than Lumineers, and are typically much healthier for the gum tissue, because they fit more intimately against the tooth. The porcelain used allows for superior color—kind of like the Old Master's techniques used in oil painting, you get layers of color that give your teeth depth and vitality.

Bonding the porcelain veneers to the teeth must be done under powerful magnification and the strictest conditions of cleanliness. We can't allow any saliva to touch the prepared porcelain as it is being bonded. If saliva contamination occurs, the bond may discolor or fail—and if it fails, the porcelain can fall off unexpectedly.

Properly done, customized veneers not only produce superior aesthetic results, but they're also longer lasting than are Lumineers. Porcelain veneers can last 10 to 15 years or more, though I'm up front with my patient about the fact that they can chip or break, and may need to be replaced sooner than a decade from now.

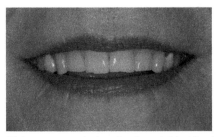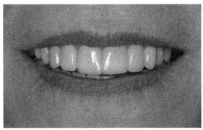

Mature woman before treatment (L); After treatment (R)

Once again, I can't stress strongly enough: To get the results you deserve, it pays to be informed. Ask the hard questions. I'm happy to provide my patients with before and after photos of *my* work—not pictures of someone else's work taken from a book or ad. In fact, you'll find plenty on my website, at www.LifeSmiles.us. I'm also more than happy to provide details of my training and experience in cosmetic dentistry. You'll find some of that on my website, but we can talk about it, too. As I noted earlier, life is about relating with other people and being able to communicate in a trusting way. I want you to be comfortable that you're working with someone you can trust.

Dental Face-Lifts: The Latest in Looking Younger

Face-lifts performed by cosmetic surgeons are considered the go-to option for looking younger these days, but their results are literally only skin-deep. Your teeth and jaws are what actually provide the underlying structure of your face, so they play a highly important role in how young (or old!) you look.

I mentioned earlier that I do restorations and cosmetic procedures on many people in their 30s whose teeth look like they're in their 90s. Just as I can take years off the look of your teeth, I can combine procedures to take years off the look of your face.

The techniques I use to achieve this are particularly useful for men and women who've lost the "vertical dimension" of the bottom part of the face. To explain what that means, let me ask you to think of how someone with dentures looks when those dentures are taken out. The only things that keep our chin from touching our nose are the teeth that are in between, so that, without them, the person looks like a witch. As the lips turn inward they disappear, and the nose comes a lot closer to the chin.

People whose teeth are all worn down can start to look 'witchy,' too. Their chin starts getting too close to their nose, and their lips turn inward. You don't see the red part of the lips (called the vermillion border) as much. And as their mouth starts to turn downward, 'marionette' creases develop at the corners, like a puppet.

Think about it: These changes occur because teeth are getting shorter, and the vertical space between the chin and nose is decreasing. That means that if we correct that shortening, then we increase that vertical space between the chin and the nose—which then corrects all those deformities that I've just described. It returns the mouth to its former shape, reverses that frowning and creasing, and brings the lips back out—even though we haven't injected the skin or the lips with fillers. This is especially appropriate for baby boomers who had four permanent premolars removed in addition to having the four wisdom teeth being removed in order to be fitted with braces. The orthodontists of that era were trained to 'make room' to bring the front teeth back and straight. We now know that was not always the best thing to do. Some of these people, as older adults, have a sunken lip profile, advanced wear on the edges or tips of the front teeth, and TMJ issues.

Often, looking younger is a bonus benefit of the dental work we're doing for structural reasons. Correcting a bad bite, putting a crown on a decayed or broken tooth, and/or fitting you with well-designed bridges, dentures, and implants can all make you look more youthful. I always take things like filling out the lips and getting the right distance between the teeth and nose into consideration when designing dentures and implants. But when a little 'lift' of youthfulness is the primary work you want done, here's my approach.

First, we'll apply the usual principles of neuromuscular dentistry: Using computer guides to measure muscles of the jaw when they're in a relaxed state, we'll determine the optimal position for the upper and lower jaws, and where the teeth should fall in between. We'll then use CAD/CAM technology to create an orthotic that restores your teeth, especially the back ones, to their original height. To do that, we'll practice what I call 'addition dentistry.'

In the past when you had a crown done on a tooth, you probably had 'subtraction dentistry.' The dentist subtracted part of your tooth by grinding around it, grinding off its top, and putting a crown down over it. When rebuilding a youthful understructure, I don't want to do subtraction dentistry. Most times the patient has already had that done, and the tooth has worn away. So instead of grinding the tooth down, I want to add to it. We do addition dentistry by bonding new tops, like little mountaintops, onto the top of the teeth.

Of course, the same basic 'addition' principles can be applied to denture wearers. We modify the design of the dentures they now wear to build the back teeth up. How long it takes to get this 'lift' simply depends on how long it takes to get a new set of cosmetically excellent dentures made. But if you still have your own teeth, I'll do my 'addition dentistry' as a process. It's a major commitment financially, and the changes you make to the teeth are permanent (in the sense that you really can't change your mind and go back to what was before). For this reason, I always like people to take their orthotic for what I call a test drive. We bond the orthotic on the lower teeth in a semi-permanent way and I ask you to wear it for one to three months. This not only ensures you like the way it makes your face look, but also ensures the new vertical dimension we've established is correct and comfortable for the joints and muscles.

In contributing to a *Wall Street Journal* article on dental facelifts, I cautioned consumers about 'overdoing' dental work for cosmetic reasons. I was quoted as noting, "You can push the envelope and get nice cosmetic results, but if you violate biological principles of health you can get in trouble." That's a quote I'm proud to stand by. If you change your bite too much, you can throw the jaw out of balance and actually cause pain. To avoid this, we'll refine the orthotic over time as you wear it and the muscles, jaw, and bite change. Once your bite is stable (i.e., it doesn't change anymore) and we're sure the jaw is in balance, we're home-free. We simply use that adjusted orthotic as our template for the porcelain crowns, then bond them permanently to your teeth.

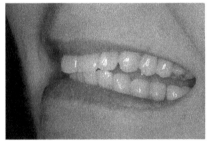 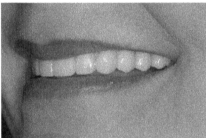

Before dental facelift (L); After (R)

MY INNER SECRET

I have a bit of a confession to make: I used to hate making the crowns I utilized in cosmetic and restorative procedures, and my patients hated them just as much. We made impressions of the mouth using gloopy putty molds that were so gross and squishy they literally made patients gag. Then I took those impressions and used them to make stone models of the actual teeth. Because the putty impressions weren't always 100 percent accurate, the models made from them weren't perfect, either. The rubber itself was challenging to work with, since it expanded and compressed at different rates from the stone. They had to be shipped out to the lab, and between the chemicals to make them, and the packaging and shipping required, the process wasn't environmentally friendly. *(continued on next page...)*

Plus, it was time consuming and inconvenient for the patient. All told, the time between taking impressions and getting crowns back would take longer than three weeks.

Inaccuracies, delays, and just plain grossness are hardly in keeping with my vision of dentistry. My patients can and should expect better from me. So I started researching better methods, and invested in CAD/CAM technology.

I've talked up CAD/CAM quite a bit already, since it's opened up a whole new era in dentistry. In my practice, it's a key component of the neuromuscular dentistry and the crowns, porcelain veneers, and implant restorations I do. But its use in making crowns is one of my favorite applications. It actually makes crafting crowns fun— both for me *and* for you.

Instead of subjecting you to gloopy, gaggy impressions and risking their inaccurate results, I now simply take a digital scan of your teeth that creates an intricate 3D image. You can actually see the image of your tooth build on the screen as we scan. It is a great way for you to participate in your care and for us to educate and inform you better. Reviewing the scan together facilitates a discussion of your wants and needs, letting us better understand the work that will be necessary to meet your goals.

The CAD/CAM system I use also allows us to fabricate crowns, veneers, and implant restorations without gooey impressions—and all the while protecting Mother Earth. Best of all, your crowns and other restorations will fit more perfectly. And because they're made of durable ceramic, they'll be extremely long lasting.

For more information on CAD/CAM technology and other state of the art technologies I use, visit
www.dentistrytoday.com/technology/1914

"Will You Remove My Silver Fillings?"

There's a short answer and a long answer to that question. The short answer is, of course, I will, if that's something you want. The longer answer requires a bit of explanation.

Fifty percent of the composition of silver fillings is mercury. Mercury is a toxic substance, so why are dentists putting it in the mouth? That's the big question. In many foreign countries, fillings containing mercury are actually outlawed or banned.

In this country, mercury is recognized as a toxic substance, but it's still allowed in the amalgam that's used to make metal fillings. If a dentist is using this type of filling, any scrap material left over must be placed into a special box that's labeled as a biohazard. If you accidentally spill some on the floor, then you have to decontaminate the whole floor area and sweep it up to put that in a special biohazard box. It has to be shipped off to be disposed of as a biohazard. But it's okay to put in your mouth? That doesn't make a whole lot of sense.

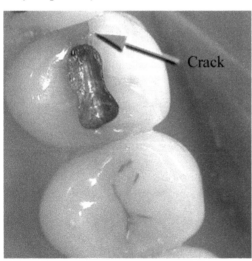

Filling and crack in tooth.

I don't use silver fillings in my practice; instead, I use tooth-colored composite resin that doesn't contain mercury. The resin fuses one side of the tooth to the other, holding it together in a way that makes it stronger. This eliminates another big drawback of those old, dark fillings. They have a lifespan of about 10 to 15 years, after which they actually corrode and puff up a bit—and when they do, the expansion can cause cracks in the teeth. In fact, that's probably one of the most common calls I get on a Monday morning. Patients will call and say, "Remember the crack you saw in that tooth? Well, it broke over the weekend."

But here's the thing: If someone comes to me and says, "I've got all these silver fillings and I think they're making me sick. Will you please drill them out and replace them?" I will tell them, "I'm not sure that's what's making you sick." I would not want to raise false hope that removing silver fillings will reverse an illness. On the other hand—and this might sound a little strange—if someone comes to me and says, "I have a mouth full of silver fillings which are ugly as hell, will you take those out and make my teeth look nice?" I say, "Sure. That's a great reason." And if you have fillings that have outlived their life expectancy and are starting to crack your teeth or corrode so you're getting cavities, that's is the best reason to have them taken out. That's the bigger danger than those silver fillings making you sick.

Toxic substances don't belong in the body, and, in rare cases, mercury fillings *can* make you sick. In an amalgam filling, the chemistry of that mercury is supposed to be bound or 'wrapped up' inside the silver so it can't leech out. And it doesn't do so immediately; it leeches out over a period of years. Some people are ultra-sensitive to its effects, and can get sick as that happens. But for most, by the time a filling is 15 years old, the mercury in it has been vaporized— you have already breathed and swallowed it and it is actually gone. So if you have a mouthful of silver fillings, you needn't freak out that you'll die if they don't come out. In an admittedly odd bit of good news, your mercury exposure is behind you by now.

CHAPTER 9

Orthodontics: Not Just for Kids

Charlene is a professor at the University of St. Thomas. Each school year, she teaches in front of hundreds of college students. Her reputation among her peers and her pupils is beyond compare. Even so, there was something that kept Charlene from even deeper engagement during her class lectures. She didn't smile as often or as wide as she knew she wanted to, because she was self-conscious about her teeth.

Charlene had two crowns done on her front teeth many years ago, and came to see me about replacing them. Not all work a dentist does can last a lifetime. Let's just say that Charlene had fared far better over the years than those two crowns.

We quickly discovered, however, that once those old crowns were replaced, Charlene would have two new beautiful front teeth that wouldn't match the rest of her smile. Basically, she'd be right back where she started. The right thing to do—and Charlene concurred after subjectively analyzing photos that we made of her teeth and smile—was to correct all the issues of the teeth that showed when she smiled. As she had already suspected, many of those issues were caused by her bad bite, which was largely to blame for the premature breakdown of her front teeth. Her treatment plan involved orthodontic repositioning of the teeth to eliminate her deep overbite, and porcelain veneers to correct the damaged teeth.

Many of my patients travel as part of their profession, so I often have to work within constrained schedules. That was the case with Charlene. I would have only five weeks from her first visit until she departed for a twelve-month sabbatical to European cities such as London, Southampton, St. Petersburg, Hamburg, Amsterdam, and Antwerp. Sacrifices of time for both Charlene and me came into play, but we found ways to mesh our schedules—as well as a clever way to get her what she wanted. We made the porcelain veneers first, then immediately delivered Invisalign® aligners that would straighten her teeth. That way, she got the impact of a beautiful smile in time for her trip, and was able to do the 'straightening' phase while traveling.

Charlene began her sabbatical with a spectacular new smile. During her trip she sent a message, along with some photos:

> I am having the time of my life and I thought you would enjoy seeing some photos of my smiling face along the way! I am delighted with my new smile—you have transformed my life in many ways with this change!

When Charlene's sabbatical is over, there's more transformation to come. She can't wait to get back up in front of a packed lecture hall to face all those students with her beautiful new smile.

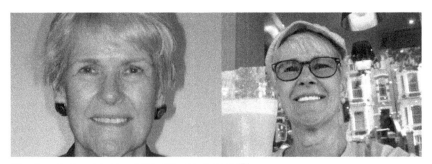

Charlene before treatment (L); After treatment (R)

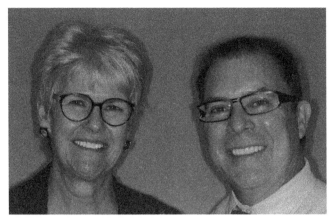

Charlene and Dr. Mitchmore

To read more about Charlene's story and to discover how orthodontics aren't just for kids visit **www.lifesmiles.us/straightenup**

Within reason, porcelain veneers can be used to give teeth a straighter, more even appearance. But when teeth are severely misaligned, the best option is orthodontics—what most people think of as 'getting braces.'

Correcting crooked teeth can make your smile more beautiful. It can also make it a lot healthier. When we fit you for orthodontic work, our goal isn't just to straighten your teeth. It's also to correct problems with your bite. Form follows function, and the functional problems created by a bad bite can increase the wear and tear on teeth, aging them fast. Sometimes, you can guess the age of a horse by looking at how worn away the teeth are. Not true with humans! I have patients in their 30s whom you would swear were 90 if you looked only at their teeth. Those teeth start looking shorter and the lower front teeth start looking thicker. Often, you can see a darker color in the center with a lighter ring around it.

Picture this: If you cut down a tree and look down at the stump, you see a ring of bark on the outside and a different color inside.

That's much like what happens to your teeth. Each tooth is covered with a shell of very hard but very brittle enamel. Enamel is whiter than the inner core of the tooth, called dentin. If you wear through the enamel, the inner dentin core of the tooth is exposed. The dentin is seven times softer than tooth enamel, so once it is exposed, it wears faster—and the enamel literally chips away because it is unsupported. If the top layer of enamel is worn and you look down on the tip of the tooth, you will see a ring of white enamel and a darker color inside that ring. If the wear is really bad, you can see a third color, like a dot, in the center. That is the nerve inside the core.

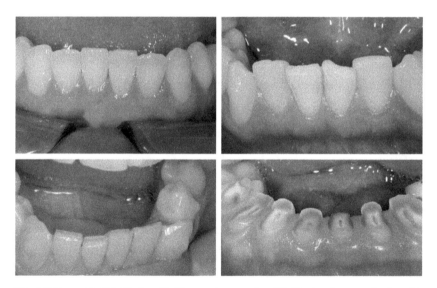

Unworn lower front teeth (top L); Very early wear (top R); Moderate wear (bottom L); Severe wear (bottom R)

Front teeth are thicker at the gum line and get thinner as you go up to the edge or tip. This means that if you cut off or wear away the tip, the biting edge of the tooth looks thicker than it did before the tooth was damaged. The nice original scalloping lines between the individual teeth are lost and the teeth look very flat or straight-across. As premature wear goes on, teeth shorten, thicken, and flatten even further, and a dark notch can develop at the gum line. As a result, your smile looks old.

Clearly, the best way to prevent such problems is to fix what caused it, your bite. One of the very best ways to do that is with the Invisalign system I use. Invisalign puts the teeth in the proper alignment so they perform better and look better. (Remember, form follows function.) But Invisalign 'braces' are far different from the ones you dreaded wearing when you were a kid. And they're not just for kids, either. I currently have patients using Invisalign who are 14 to 78 years old!

When you and I were kids, you went to the orthodontist and got braces that gave us a mouthful of metal bands and wires. We went in periodically and had our braces 'tightened'; basically, they were crunched down on our teeth until they hurt. Gradually that forced our teeth—and hopefully our bite—back into proper alignment. These days, Invisalign provides a much better method. Using CAD/CAM technology, we design a series of thin plastic aligners for you to wear. We actually produce a CAD/CAM artist's rendition of what your teeth look like now, and what they're going to look like a year from now. The aligners are then designed to be worn in an order that places only gentle pressure on your teeth, gradually guiding them back into place.

The aligners themselves are much like ultra-thin bleaching trays; the thickness of a couple sheets of paper, they fit over the teeth right up to the gum line. They work great. You don't have to worry about popping wires or missing brackets. And because you take them off to thoroughly clean your teeth, you don't have to worry about getting spinach caught in them or having dark marks on your teeth when all is said and done. The trick is it that the pressure applied by Invisalign has to be almost continuous, so they have to stay in your mouth about 20 out of 24 hours of the day.

I am one of the few dentists in the world who has actually trained at the Invisalign technical center in Costa Rica. My first-hand knowledge of the design process allows me to be certified to use the latest generation of aligner material called Smart Track. Smart Track has only recently been introduced. It is more flexible and is a real step forward in making orthodontic corrections happen quickly, predictably, and comfortably. The material gives your tooth a 3D hug that can move it in any direction that I design.

When you're going through the Invisalign treatment, we want to make sure your teeth alignment is progressing according to the plan. To do that, you'll come in about every six to eight weeks. And while Invisalign's cost is a bit higher than conventional 'metal-mouth' braces, it actually works faster. Of course, the total length of time you'll wear them depends on how much correction you need. Some very minor corrections may take as few as five aligners and only ten weeks of time. Some major corrections can take more than 26 aligners and two years of time. But on average, Invisalign can do in a year what metal braces take several years to do. Most busy professionals appreciate the time savings, not to mention Invisalign's look. They really are nearly invisible to the eye.

CHAPTER TEN

The Boomerang Effect: Why Dentistry Is My Life Mission

"The game of life is a game of boomerangs. Our thoughts, deeds, and words return to us sooner or later, with astounding accuracy."
—FLORENCE SHINN

Suzanne may have escaped from the nightmare of domestic violence, but a reminder greeted her each morning when she looked in the mirror.

For 12 years, she had been living with a broken front tooth. Even though she had moved on to rebuild a life for herself and her two sons, she rarely smiled. If she did, she knew what people would see. That hesitance to smile became a barrier to building the future of what she dreamed—for her children and for herself. Job opportunities seemed to slip just beyond her grasp. A solid social network of friends seemed nearly impossible to assemble. Suzanne knew the signs of depression, and she knew she needed to overcome it.

When Suzanne came to see me, she actually already had beautiful teeth. Her general health was very good and her oral hygiene was excellent. Unfortunately, like many people who go for extended periods of time without professional dental cleanings, she had moderate periodontal disease—some buildup of hard tartar under the gum with resultant inflammation. Her teeth were yellowed from age and the core of the tooth was being exposed.

And yes, her upper-right front tooth had an obvious broken, ragged edge. Just talking about it took some of the light out of Suzanne's eyes, and it was disheartening to watch her lose so much vibrancy simply by turning her attention to this reminder of a life she wanted to leave behind. Her left front tooth was slightly chipped, as well. I didn't have any doubt that if we could just turn back the clock on her smile, she'd begin to see some positive changes.

Which is exactly what happened. Over a two-week period, we cleared up the gum disease with the Gums of Steel program. That involved a deep cleaning, coaching on how to remove daily biofilm build-up at home, and special mouthwashes, brushes, and diet aids. Next was to whiten the teeth. Then I turned my attention to that broken front tooth.

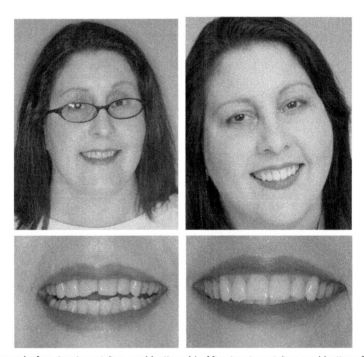

Suzanne before treatment (top and bottom L); After treatment (top and bottom R)

I'll let Suzanne describe what happened when we handed her a mirror to see her repaired tooth:

> *I smiled, and when I saw that smile, I cried. At that moment*
> *I realized that I had forgotten how to really smile—a true*
> *one given from the heart. This realization was profound.*
> *I also realized that my youngest child had never seen that*
> *from me.*

Broken teeth are easy for me to fix. Broken lives are a different story. One thing that was not broken about Suzanne was her determination. Fixing her smile repaired her ability to utilize the psychological and emotional strength she always had within herself, but didn't feel worthy of bringing forth.

Soon after we fixed Suzanne's smile, she stopped by with her children to say hello. I asked her how things were going for her. "You helped me to again be the person I really am," she said to me. "There was always this happy, outgoing and productive person in me. Thanks for helping me find her again."

To read more about Suzanne's story and to give yourself a smile evaluation visit **www.lifesmiles.us/ratemysmile**

As I've told you, I am grateful for the life I've been given. Despite the hard lessons I've learned, I'm grateful for what life has taught me. And I'm supremely grateful for the gift I've been given by being a dentist—because to me, it's not just a profession, but it is absolutely a gift. Being a dentist has allowed me to be a part of so many life-changing transformations. Time and again, I've seen embarrassed, self-conscious, even downright broken, people turn to confident, happy, smiling people.

I am constantly blessed to be a part of that. And I've always felt strongly that it's my duty to give back to my profession, and to my community, in return for all the goodness I have received. Professionally, I have lectured at dental meetings to teach dentists what I do, and authored many dental articles. One of my proudest accomplishments was being chosen to serve as Chairman of the Board of Trustees for the American Academy of Cosmetic Dentistry Charitable Foundation for two terms.

Personally, I've also reached out to others through causes that are near and dear to me. I have used my non-profit and political experiences to serve on the Board of Directors of Bering Omega, a group devoted to people infected and affected by HIV during the crisis years of the epidemic. The Texas Legislature appointed me a Trustee to the newly created Montrose Management District, a political body that makes assessments on commercial property and uses that money for the betterment of the district where I live and work. But some of the most fulfilling work I do is for the Give Back A Smile program, a nationwide network of volunteer dentists who restore smiles to victims of domestic violence or intimate domestic partner abuse, free of charge.

Give Back A Smile

When I first became a member of the American Academy of Cosmetic Dentistry, I considered its Give Back A Smile™ (GBAS) program an excellent humanitarian cause. I decided to become a GBAS volunteer dentist and hold a 'Whitening Day' at my office, donating my proceeds to the program. The whitening day went well and I was soon assigned a case.

Little did I know how near and dear this cause would become to me. Domestic violence was already causing pain and destruction very close to home: My own sister, Laura, was a silent victim. Laura was

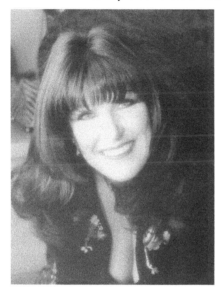

beautiful, smart, hardworking, and the loving mother of three children. By every outward indication, she was extremely successful. I had no idea whatsoever how dreadful things were for her behind closed doors. Unfortunately, I never learned that until it was too late. My sister was not a domestic violence survivor; ultimately, it ended her life by suicide. I could not save my sister's life, but for her I can help save the lives of others. I now dedicate my work for Give Back a Smile to Laura's memory.

One in every four women—that's 25 percent of all women—are victims of domestic violence (http://www.ncadv.org/files/Domesti cViolenceFactSheet%28National%29.pdf). They are our mothers, our sisters, our aunts, and our daughters. Members of Give Back a Smile have donated more than $8 million in services to women, and men, who have survived domestic violence. I'm proud to be among these dentists. Every patient we touch through this program is not only a smile saved, but it is truly a life saved. How do I know that? I've been told so by the patients themselves—woman like Suzanne, and like Tina.

Tina loved to laugh, and sing Gospel music in her church choir. But after the one-two punch of losing her home in Galveston to a hurricane, then losing her front teeth to domestic violence, she didn't laugh or sing. She was jobless and living in a shelter for battered women when a social worker told her about Give Back A Smile program. She filled out an application for the program and I took on her case.

The Give Back A Smile program provided Tina with a travel voucher to get from Galveston to Houston, and while she was delighted to come to my office, she was clearly tentative and nervous. Once we restored her smile, however, she went from bashful to beaming. And within a few weeks of returning to Galveston, she had a reliable job.

On the one year anniversary of having her smile restored, I called Tina to ask how she was doing. She was so excited that I had called, and told me that she is now smiling all the time. "People don't believe it is me when I show them the before and after pictures you gave me," she said. "But I tell them, it really is me!"

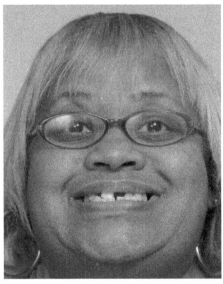 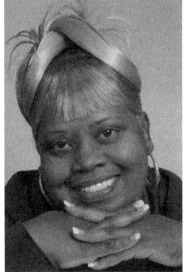

Tina before treatment (L); After treatment (R)

Would I win any awards for the work I did on Tina? In terms of professional or clinical awards, I have no idea. But the results that Tina got meant more to me than any award I've received in my field. She is living proof of the Give Back a Smile motto: Restore a Smile, Restore a Life.

A Life of Daily Miracles

Being a dentist has allowed me to restore the lives of women such as Suzanne and Tina, but it's also blessed me on a daily basis through the patients I see regularly. It's allowed me to help the child who could eat corn through a picket fence become a handsome, successful young man. It's allowed me to help the mother who's spent her life tending to others finally give herself permission to get what *she* deserves. My patients are amazing people, as you can tell by some of their 'Cinderella' stories.

Willie

Willie had a heart transplant a number of years ago that gave him a second chance on life. He was so grateful for that second chance that he began to work as a volunteer, talking with patients who are need of a heart transplant. He speaks with them and their families about what to expect from a transplant, and how his own transplant changed his life.

Willie is a truly wonderful person whose smile did not reflect his inner light. He had missing teeth, and those that remained were crooked. He wasn't only embarrassed about the ugly appearance of his smile, but he was also concerned that it was interfering with his own mission. He knew that sometimes his life-changing message was not getting across, because people would stare at his ugly smile and dismiss what he was saying.

Through the generosity of an anonymous donor and a matching contribution by my office, Willie is getting the smile he deserves. The gift of a smile will enable him to touch many more people and share with them the gift of a second heart. This is the message that Willie sent me on the day of his dental implant surgery:

Hello Dr. Mitchmore,

Thank you for such a great and non-painful dental procedure today. Today has given me my entire life back. My heart transplant and now a new smile so the world can see just how happy and blessed I am. You and your staff are so professional at what you do and with the biggest smile on your face at all times.

I knew when I walked in and saw how happy everyone in your office was that I wanted what you all had, that smile and joyful attitude I saw and felt as I enter the world of LIFESMILES.

By the way I forgot to get my teeth from you so I can put them under my pillow for the TOOTH FAIRY (SMILE!!!),

Please thank everybody at LIFESMILES for a job well done.

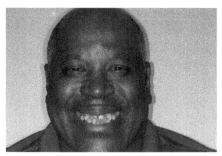 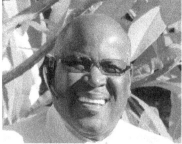

Willie before treatment (L); After treatment (R)

Cathy

When I first met Cathy, she had been living with Grave's disease for two years—but she'd been living with poor dental health for most of her life. Cathy is not a victim of domestic violence but hers is a story of transformation from how her dental problems and dental treatment gave her a feeling similar to that of abuse. A string of negative experiences with dentists had left her afraid to seek regular care; as a result, she had lost all but a few of her upper teeth, and wore a six-tooth bridge with a partial denture attached. Cathy was scheduled for a thyroidectomy (surgical removal of her thyroid to treat her Graves' disease) when she was brushing her teeth one morning and heard a loud 'clink.' To her horror, the bridge that had been cemented into her mouth for 10 years had fallen out, and lay in the sink.

Cathy was devastated, and cried like a baby—then hit the computer to find a dentist who might help her quickly, since her surgery was only a few days away. Googling "Best dentist in Houston" pulled up my practice, and she called my office immediately. As for what happened next, I'll let Cathy tell you in her own words:

It must have been fate, because the nice lady on the other end of the phone told me that the office was closed, but they were doing some remodeling and the staff was there packing and cleaning. 'Janie' could hear how embarrassed and overwhelmed I was and was so kind and caring. She said if I didn't mind that they weren't professionally dressed, she would certainly like to help me out and to come on in.

When I got there I will say, I was beside myself, but Janie and Dr. Mitchmore's staff put my mind at ease and placed my bridge back in temporarily. We spoke at length about my dental history and possible options, took x-rays and pictures, and prepared me to meet Dr. Mitchmore once my surgery was completed. I was deathly afraid that my bridge would come out while getting anesthesia during my surgery but Janie assured me that if it did, she would personally come to the hospital and help me. Who does that in this day and time??!! I have never met such caring, professional, detail-oriented dental office staff in my life!

As it turned out, Janie did a great job, because my bridge didn't come out during surgery but knowing I could count on Dr. Mitchmore's staff eased my mind tremendously and that was only the beginning...

So now it's my return visit to meet Dr. Mitchmore. My first instinct about Dr. Mitchmore was how kind he was and what a genuinely compassionate human being he is. You know from the moment you meet him that he cares. He is gracious and understanding, generous and patient. He is warm, talented, and passionate for his craft. His chair-side manner is unequaled and in my opinion his skill unsurpassed by any other dentist. My current dental plan is vast and includes full upper implants, lower braces, extractions, etc. I'm on phase one to restore my mouth to better health. I now have temporary teeth on my new implants and I can't even begin to describe what it feels like to not have to put a metal partial into my mouth every day the sun comes up!!! Even my temporary teeth have made such a positive change in my life. I can't wait to see the final results!!! As extremely nervous as I was to get started, Dr. Mitchmore and his staff have totally changed my viewpoint about seeing the dentist. I no longer fear my appointments and have definitely found "my" dentist. Thank you so much to Dr. Mitchmore and his fantastic team for being the best dental team in Houston! God bless you all!

James

James is a good man making his own way in the world. He did not have the benefit of a traditional family as a boy, and got his education from the University of Hard Knocks on the streets of Houston. He made a few mistakes along the way, but now works very hard as a sound and lighting technician for a production company. He has been a dependable employee for many years, and is well liked by the owner and his co-workers.

When James first came to my office, he talked with no expression, and would not allow anyone to see him laugh or smile. He covered mouth with his hand while talking because his teeth were unsightly and embarrassing to him. I quickly found James to be a very friendly person. But his body language could easily lead others to perceive him as distant or unapproachable.

Almost immediately after I greeted James, he told me that he knew all of his teeth would need to be removed, and that someone was going to help him pay for it. I listened politely; I've heard this self-diagnosis before, and often find the situation is not as bad as the patient fears. But after only a brief look at James, I knew he was right. I also knew there was no need to review pictures of his teeth on a large monitor and embarrass him further, especially since he was already fighting back tears. I invited him to talk to me about his plans.

James told me that his boss's wife had recently died, and from that loss he was to receive a special gift. James's boss and his wife had both appreciated James's hard work and great attitude, so his boss decided that one way to honor his wife would be to use part of her estate to get a new smile for James. I was incredibly moved by that, and invited James to bring his boss to his treatment planning consultation.

His boss came in and we agreed on a plan of action to cover all of James's dental costs. One of his boss's friends (whom James had never even met) also offered to chip in. James contributed as well, by doing the sound and lighting at a benefit for Give Back a Smile, and at a party that launched this book. Once all plans were in place, James's teeth were removed under IV Sedation, and he received the smile of his dreams. There were lots of tears of joy on that day!

A few weeks later, James arrived at my office with a thank-you gift of a homemade chocolate amaretto cheesecake. He said he'd recently been one of 400 people attending a celebration of life party for his boss's wife. There, he'd met his boss's friend—the one who had helped him—as well as many other people, who told him how great he looked. He told me he felt incredibly blessed, happy, and grateful. Then I noticed the shirt James was wearing, and knew that I had to ask him to take a picture with me. In that picture, I'm smiling and holding a delicious cheesecake. James's smiling and wearing a T-shirt that says "Brand New Me."

The thanks I receive from my patients never fail to touch me deeply. They are powerful illustrations of what I call the Boomerang Effect: Being a dentist allows me to pay it forward for the gifts I've been given—and by giving back, I receive priceless gifts in return.

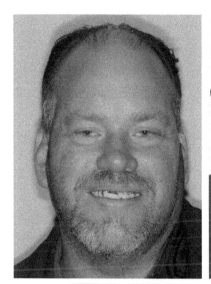
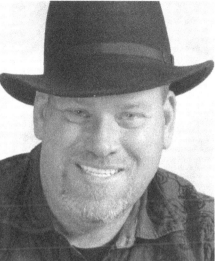
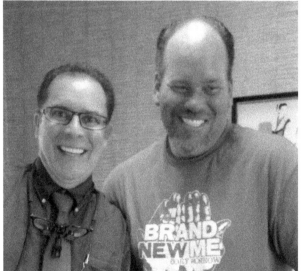

Jamie before treatment (top L); After treatment (top R and bottom)

CHAPTER ELEVEN

Your Own Life of Smiles: Getting the Journey Started

I wrote this book because dentistry is my mission. I've shared my personal struggles with you because I want to fulfill that mission by being a ray of hope for others. I want to serve as proof that, like me, you can emerge from darkness. Life has taught that living with secrets can be damaging—and dentistry has taught me that too many people are harboring secrets about their smiles. Thankfully, I've also learned that by letting go of our secrets, we can be set free and embrace the best of life. I want you to learn that, too. I want you to know that no matter what obstacles you face, you can overcome them and get the rewards you so richly deserve.

When it comes to getting the dental care they deserve, however, there's one last secret that holds people back: Often, they simply don't know where to start. Let's jump that final hurdle now.

If you're in the Houston area, you can start by checking out the LifeSmiles website, www.LifeSmiles.us, or even giving my office a call. My staff can discuss your personal situation with you over the phone in a caring and respectful way, and you can come in for an initial consultation. But if you're not in the Houston area, or just aren't ready to make a call, I'd like to get you started on your journey today with some user-friendly self-tests and checklists I've developed.

Getting What You Need: The Traffic-Light Test

The Dental Traffic Light test is a self-test I developed to help you determine where your dental health stands, and how much work you may need. Modeled after work done at the Kois Center in Seattle, it's pretty simple to take. All you need to do is answer 'yes' or 'no' to the following questions. Be honest! And if you're not sure of an answer, it's probably a 'yes.' Then tally up your 'yes' answers and refer to the traffic light colors listed below.

	Y	N
GUMS (PERIODONTAL) QUESTIONS		
Have you ever been diagnosed with gum disease?		
Do you have gum recession?		
Any blood relatives with gum disease?		
Have you ever noticed an unpleasant odor in your mouth?		
Do you smoke?		
Are your teeth becoming loose or shifting?		
BIOMECHANICAL QUESTIONS		
Have you had any new cavities within the past 3 years?		
Do you have a dry mouth?		
Any teeth sensitive to hot, cold, biting or sweets?		
Do you avoid brushing any part of your mouth		
Do you feel or notice any holes or cavities in your teeth?		
Do you drink more than 2 sodas/week?		
Not counting wisdom teeth, are you missing more than one tooth?		

BITE AND JAW JOINT QUESTIONS		
Do you have problems chewing gum?		
Do you have problems chewing bagels or hard foods?		
Have your teeth changed in the last five years, become shorter, thinner, worn?		
Are your teeth crowding or developing spaces?		
Do you have more than one bite?		
Do you wake up with an awareness of your teeth or sore face muscles?		
Do you have muscle tension headaches?		
Ever worn a bite appliance/night guard?		
Do your joints pop, crack, grate? Do you have a limited mouth opening?		
SKELETAL–FACIAL/TOOTH FEATURES QUESTIONS		
Are your teeth in what you feel is an ideal position?		
Are you self-conscious about your teeth?		
Have you ever been disappointed with previous dental work?		
Is there anything about the appearance of your teeth that you would like to change?		
Total		

If your "Yes" score is: **Your Dental Traffic Light is:**

0–4   Green

5–18   Yellow

19–26   Red

If your score is 'Green,' you are one of those fortunate individuals who is going to have very few dental problems! Your dental visits will be quick and easy, and your dental bills will be low.

If your score is 'Yellow,' you are in the majority of patients. That means you and your dentist and hygienist need to be friends! You have risk factors that make you prone to some dental problems. If you stay on top of dental issues before they get out of hand or painful, your dental experiences can be pleasant, even if it is not your favorite past time. You will have some ongoing needs and expenses. These can be kept to a minimum with regular care. Going at things this way is always cheaper than waiting until something breaks or hurts. As you know, yellow lights can turn into red lights.

If your score is 'Red,' you and your dentist need to be really close friends. This is someone that has quite a few issues stacked up against them; it is going to take a lot of continuing care to achieve dental health. If you're in the 'Red' zone, you may be faced with significant dental bills. Restoring your dental health will require an investment, but it's an investment that's definitely worthwhile—and it's far superior to the alternative. You know the penalties are steep if you run a red light! If you keep ignoring your dental issues, the results can be catastrophic.

Getting What You Want: Five Mistakes NOT to Make When Selecting a Dentist

Many people really don't know what they want in terms of dental care, because they don't know what they *can* have. When it comes to choosing a dental provider, you can have it all—knowledge, experience, a caring team and environment, excellent value, and good customer service. But you can't have it unless you ask for it. Far too many times, people who are really in search of excellence go about their own way of screening a dentist by asking all the wrong questions and looking at all the wrong things. Here's a primer on how to correct some top mistakes.

Mistake #1. Asking "Do you take my insurance?" This is an important question. Is it really the most important question to ask first? No. Insurance is a deciding factor for some, but it really should be the last question that you ask when searching out the perfect dentist for you. An interesting fact dental insurance companies do not want you to know: *In the State of Texas* (and in this state only, thanks to strong dental insurance laws) you do not have to go to 'in network' providers. Your policy may talk about 'in network' and 'out of network' providers, but you'll get benefits either way!

Mistake #2. Assuming the dentists on the 'Preferred Provider List' are the better dentists. WRONG! Greedy insurance companies have clever ways of misleading people. One would think that 'preferred' somehow indicates these are better-than-average dentists. You'd assume that the insurance company checked credentials, reviewed competency, skills, and cleanliness of the office. Not the case. 'Preferred' simply means the insurance company 'prefers' the dentists on this list because they will pay out the least and make the company the most profit. It is absolutely no indication of a good dentist—and, unfortunately, it's sometimes an indication of just the opposite.

Mistake #3. Nothing is hurting. I do not need to go to the dentist. When you were a kid, the reason you went to the dentist was to fix cavities. As an adult, the main reason to go to the dentist and have

THE GIFT OF A LIFE SMILE

your teeth cleaned is to have healthy gums. That's what holds your teeth in place! If you wait till something hurts, you waste a lot of time, money, and preventable pain.

Mistake #4. Doing only what insurance pays for. If you are fortunate enough to have some type of dental insurance, shouldn't that be viewed as assistance to get the level of dental health that you truly want or deserve? Unfortunately, it's not. 'Dental insurance' is another bad example of clever words. It should not be called insurance at all. It is not catastrophic insurance like medical insurance in any way. It is really just an annual contract that will pay out a set dollar amount per year (typically $1,500—and that has not gone up in 30 years!). It is not at all based upon what you might need or want.

Mistake #5. "I will just wait and have them all taken out and get implants." We discussed this earlier in the book, but I mention it again here because I don't want you procrastinating—or choosing a dentist whose first idea is to remove, then replace, all your teeth with implants. I love the wonderful world of dental implants that I do. They are a fabulous answer for someone who simply *must* lose one or more teeth. But it is both cheaper and better to have the real thing, and keep your natural teeth, if you can. You really need to be careful about quick-to-act dentists who offer one-size-fits-all strategies, like 'All on four" and 'A Smile in One Day.' Often, they make removing your natural teeth, rather than working to save them, sound like a quick and easy fix. It isn't, believe me.

Getting What You Deserve: 10 Things You Must Know When Choosing a Dentist

As proud as I am of my practice, I need to be honest, as usual. There's no such thing as a perfect dentist. What you should be seeking—and can, indeed, find—is the dentist who's perfect for you. To my mind, that's one who is kind and caring, non-judgmental, and someone you can trust. Just as importantly, it's someone with excellent credentials, strong clinical experience, and a commitment to keeping up with both state-of-the-art technology and advancement of their skills. Only 1 to 3 percent of professionals like dentists, lawyers, architects, and engineers are true Masters in their field. Only 5 to 10 percent are excellent, another 5 to 10 percent are above average, and 20 to 30 percent are average. That means that 50 percent are BELOW average. Which category are you comfortable with? I think you deserve the best. If you think so too, here are the big questions to consider—along with the answers that indicate you've found the dentist you deserve:

1. **What do actual patients say about the dentist and the office?** How can you find out? If you have not been personally referred to the dentist, I advise going to your computer to Google the dentist you're considering, and then clicking on the 'Google reviews.' This will show you what actual patients have said about their experience there. Google is one of the best sources of accurate independent reviews, because the dentist cannot 'stack the deck' with lots of phony or solicited reviews. Google has strict rules and filters on weeding out spam or fake reviews. The dentist also cannot pay Google to take away bad reviews.

2. **Does the dentist have experience?** Experience is important, because no dentist learns everything he or she needs to know by 'just' going to dental school. The fact is that dental schools have difficulty fitting all of the basic science, medicine, pharmacology, and anatomy into their four-year curriculum. They're hard-pressed for time to teach dental techniques, materials, and technology. Dental students practice on models, then on a few live patients to learn most types of dental procedures—but certainly not all. So even the brightest and most well-meaning new dentist has not seen all of the unusual versions of dental problems or performed much beyond truly basic procedures. Experience is one of those things that you do not appreciate until you have it. That is true in most all aspects of life. Experience means time to mature, and gives quiet confidence and ease. That is why any professional sports player, actor, dancer, or musician makes their craft look easy or effortless. They have practiced and stumbled over that very same stroke, step, line, or song over and over and over until it is perfect and looks easy. Dentistry is the same way. To find out how much experience your dentist has, poke around his or her website. Look for examples of the dentist's actual work—not stock pictures that are 'borrowed.' See if the dentist has written stories or articles about their work. See if there is a variety of advanced services offered beyond the basic fillings, crowns, veneers, root canals, and cleanings. Some will tell you they have more than so many years of experience, but that does not guarantee they've improved their skills and techniques over those years. While one dentist can spend 20 years learning and growing each

year, another can spend the same 20 years repeating their first year over and over, without ending up much improved.

3. **Does the dentist have good teeth?** You might be thinking that is a crazy statement. Consider this: Would you go to a personal fitness trainer who is out of shape? Would you go to a physician who has poor health habits? Would you go to a lawyer who seldom wins a case? I find it appalling when I go to dental meetings and see how many dentists have neglected their own teeth to a point that is noticeable at a conversational distance away. I personally find it hypocritical to provide advice and treatment if you are not taking care of your own teeth. To a patient, it should be downright scary. Look at the people who work in the office. Do they take dentistry seriously in their own mouth? Do they and their friends and family have their dental work done by the dentist they work for?

Just because I am a dentist does not mean that I am immune from dental problems. I was a fat little boy who loved caramel squares wrapped in clear plastic. I had a mouth full of cavities. I currently have one root canal filling from my brother Glenn throwing a spoon that hit a front tooth. I had full old-fashioned wire braces when I was 37 years old. I have 10 porcelain crowns and 10 Porcelain veneers. Those were done a long time ago and are serving me very well, as well as a couple of gold foil fillings that were done in my mouth while I was in dental school. Every time I sit in the dental chair to have dental treatment done, it always makes me a better and more caring dentist.

4. **Does the dentist run on time for appointments?** It is a matter of respect to run on time. Your time should be considered as important as anyone else's. Of course, there can be a truly unusual circumstance or emergency that puts a dentist off-schedule, but that should be rare. Constantly running late for appointments can be a sign of disorganization, lack of leadership and training, or greed (from packing too many patients in). Or it could signify that this dentist simply doesn't care.

5. **Is the office clean?** It is not enough to assume that instruments and rooms are clean and properly disinfected. It's a dental office, so germ control is extremely important. How can you get a good idea of a dentist's attitude toward cleanliness? My secret tip is to look in the bathroom. If it is trashy and anything less than spotless, that could be a clue as to how the clinical part of the office is maintained. Personally, I'd be outta there. And even if the bathroom passes inspection, be sure to ask questions about how the dentist sterilizes instruments. Ideally, it should involve using ultrasonics as well as an autoclave.

6. **Is the dentist thorough?** A new patient's initial examination should be like a physical examination conducted by a physician. It should include a health history to see if there are any medical conditions that could have dental implications. Also, some conditions, like a heart murmur with regurgitation, or heart valve disease, or recent artificial joint replacements, require taking an antibiotic before having dental treatment. Diabetes must also be taken into account,

as it creates special concern for patients with gum infections. Other questions the patient should consider: Does the dentist evaluate the condition of the muscles and joints of the face? Is there a thorough examination for gum disease and a screen for oral cancer? Is there a thorough evaluation of existing or old fillings and crowns? Are diagnostic-quality X-rays and photographs made? Is there a discussion of your risk factors and your goals for your teeth? All of these answers should be 'yes.' This type of in-depth dental physical can take almost an hour. It simply cannot be done in a typical 10-minute 'check up.'

7. **Is the dentist gentle?** The three things that concern people the most about dental care are: (1) Is it going to hurt? (2) How much does it cost? and (3) How does it look? A gentle dentist will be known for his or her gentleness. There should be only minor discomfort after most dental treatment. During dental treatment, the process should be virtually pain free. Gums should not be bleeding after having fillings, crowns, root canals, or veneers done. You should not feel like your head is being jerked around or stretched in multiple directions. Is the dentist sympathetic if you say something is uncomfortable and stops to address it? Does the dentist or staff offer sedation? There are different levels of sedation. The best sedation is IV Sedation, which requires very advanced skills and certification.

8. **Is the dentist current on the latest dental breakthroughs?** The state requires a minimum of 12 hours of continuing education each year. Better dentists will routinely have more

than 100 hours of continuing education per year. They will have extensive hands-on training at advanced dental institutes, not just weekend seminars at hotels. Look for recognition of advanced training through certificates on dentists' walls or websites, naming institutes like Pankey Institute, Kois or FACE, the Las Vegas Institute for Advanced Dental Studies, and the Dawson Institute. You want a dentist who is up to date on the wonderful technology that is now available. It makes for higher-quality dental treatment that fits better, looks better, and lasts longer.

9. **Is the dentist a member of dental organizations and charity minded?** Membership in various dental associations and charities indicate the dentist is a good community member or leader. Involvement in charities indicates a sense of citizenship, gratitude, and compassion.

10. **Does the dental office ask about your insurance first?** While insurance is an important assistance for many people, I believe this is the last question to be dealt with by a dental office. The nine questions above are criteria that *must* be met, regardless of insurance. If the dental office is more concerned about your dental insurance than what your needs and concerns are, it could be an indication that the dentist is focused more on money than on people. Dental insurance is sadly very misunderstood these days. People are beginning to realize that it really is not insurance at all; it is merely a contract for a small amount of help with dental expenses. Even if you need an extensive amount of dental work, dental insurance will typically pay to have only one or two teeth restored per

year. It is contract-based on a maximum number of dollars—usually around $1,500—paid out annually. As I mentioned before, that amount has not gone up significantly in 30 years! Again and again, I see patients who are very disappointed when they learn how little dental insurance pays. They usually hear that certain procedures are covered 50 percent or 80 percent or even 100 percent. What they don't know is that the insurance payout is capped and pays no more once that low cap of around $1,500 is paid, no matter how much dentistry is needed or done.

Bonus question: What does your gut say? The mouth is a very personal part of your body. It is important that you entrust it to someone *you* can trust. Your dentist shouldn't just be someone who tells you what to do—he or she should be someone with whom you can establish a relationship, and work with in a team effort to enhance your oral health and your life. When finding someone as important as this, your gut instinct can serve as a valuable guide.

INFECTION PROTECTION: A CRITICAL CONCERN

There was horrible news out of Tulsa, Oklahoma, in 2013. The headlines read that 7,000 patients of a Tulsa dentist are being tested to see if they got any infections from dirty instruments. It should never have happened. He was an oral surgeon who had more extensive training in hospital-grade sterile procedures than general dentists receive. There is simply no excuse.

I was shocked at the news, but the media did a valuable service in making it public. These sorts of behaviors should be exposed, so that the bad guys can be ousted and the public better informed.

The chatter that came down the wire inside the dental profession said that this guy was ignoring all standard protocols on basic sanitation, much less sterile technique. What really bothers me is that he had an office full of employees who should also have known better. If reports are correct, they were basically as bad as the guy in charge. Apparently, this dentist was using the same vials of medicine on different people, and instead of running instruments through a steam autoclave (a special sterilizing machine you'll learn more about below), he and his staff were disinfecting instruments with bleach. The problem: Bleach makes instruments corrode or rust—and germs love to live in corrosion and rust. Evidently the autoclave that they did use on some instruments was not tested, and was not functioning properly at killing all germs and spores.

The dentist was exposed when a few previously healthy people in Tulsa got sick, and doctors could not find an obvious reason. Just as occurs in food-poisoning incidents, investigators had to be detectives and start piecing together clues to find a common element among the people who were sick. The evidence pointed to one thing all had shared: They had seen the same oral surgeon. Of course, this made for a sensational story and I condemn the surgeon's actions as they were reported. I do want to clarify that 7,000 people were not infected; there were a very few. At last word, authorities were asking 7,000 former patients who were apparently healthy to *voluntarily* undergo testing for infectious diseases. Still, this story illustrates how improper sterilization techniques can put you at risk.

There is an enormous difference between disinfection and sterilization. I like to use going to a restaurant as an example. We use silverware and glasses that go into our mouth, potentially leaving germs on those utensils. I feel completely safe if that restaurant washes the dishes with soap and hot water before I use those same utensils. Those utensils have been disinfected. They were not exposed to blood. However, you could not do surgery with those utensils. That is because when you do surgery, skin is cut open, instruments go inside and under the skin, and then the skin is sewed up. ANY germs or spores introduced deep inside could grow, fester, and become an infection. Also, any germs that were inside the flesh could be passed on to the instruments. Germs such as hepatitis are not killed with just soap and water. (Interestingly the most publically feared germ—the one that causes HIV—is easily killed by soap and water. Hepatitis is the one that professionals are really worried about.) Hepatitis and similar germs and spores are killed in a machine called a 'steam autoclave.' An autoclave is a metal chamber kind that looks like an expensive pressure cooker. The instruments are subjected to high heat, steam, and pressure, and the combination kills any germs known to man.

Here is our standard procedure in the field of dentistry, and the one I use with instruments: First, they are rinsed and cleaned. Then, they go into an ultrasonic cleaner with enzymes to completely clean and disinfect them. Then, they are placed into special pouches or bags and sealed. Then, that pouch is processed in an autoclave.

We are required to place a test tablet in the autoclave on a regular basis. That test tablet is then sent to an independent laboratory to make certain the autoclave is up to specs and kills all germs. It seems this oral surgeon in Tulsa did not do that. Purely by coincidence, at about the same time this story hit the news, my office invested more than $18,000 in upgrading to larger autocalves and ultrasonic baths to handle our growing demand. These are important behind-the-scenes activities that usually go unnoticed by patients, but are critical to providing them with the highest level of care.

So what can you do to feel safe going to the dentist? Use your built-in crap detectors! When you go in the office, does it look, feel, and smell really clean? If not, cleanliness is not the priority it should be—and sterilizing instruments may not be a priority, either. And do not hesitate to ask the dentist up front if he or she follows the sterilization procedures I've outlined above. It's entirely OK to ask. You have the right to know.

As a member of our LifeSmiles' Family, you receive our unconditional satisfaction guarantee. As professionals, we stand behind the quality of our work. If one of our services, in part or in full, does not meet your satisfaction and leave you a Raving Fan of LifeSmiles, we will do everything in our power to remedy the issue and put a smile back on your face.

An Ever-Brightening Future

The field of dentistry is expanding rapidly these days, and it's exciting to be a part of that. It's even more exciting to look at what the future of dentistry might be. Today, much of the dentistry is done like an artist or architect wielding a pencil on paper. It's free-hand. When we're picking up a drill or a scalpel and wielding it in the mouth, that's free-hand. With what I know about advancements going on in CAD/CAM technology and computer-guided techniques, I foresee a future in which dentistry is guided more and more robotically, with more precision than we can achieve free-hand.

The other big area that will brighten the future of dentistry is bioengineering. We use some of it today—healing aids such as platelet-rich plasma and platelet-rich fibrinogen are breakthroughs in bioengineering. But dental science is doing some truly exciting work in other areas: Using donated bone and donated skin to actually grow new tissue both in the laboratory and directly in the mouth, even stimulating part of the tooth itself to grow.

I'm not threatened by that future in any way; I embrace it. I know it will require dentists to have an even higher degree of skills. We've got to be smart enough to use that technology, and use it to optimal result. And we've got to provide the artistry behind any procedure that uses it. I'm totally up for those tasks.

I'm excited about the future in dentistry. I'm excited at what it can do for you. But what I'm most excited about is the new future you can begin now. Isn't it time to rid yourself of the dirty secrets or nagging worry you're keeping about your mouth?

READY TO TEST YOUR SMILE IQ?

A well-informed dental patient makes the best decisions—and now that you've read this book, you're much better prepared to make the decision that's right for you. But to test your knowledge and learn even more, I've developed a series of fun, true/false quizzes you can take by simply surfing to www.lifesmiles.us/IQ. Hope you enjoy them—and I hope that the knowledge you gain from them, and from this book, motivates you to investigate your own bright future. I'm more than happy to have you visit my office so we can explore that future together.

THE LIFESMILES EXPERIENCE

LifeSmiles is the embodiment of ideal dentistry. With the use of advanced technology that is powered by the aesthetic eye, we create confident smiles, while minimizing pain. This is accomplished with friendliness, excellence in performance, and thoughtful sensitivity to the feelings and concerns of all our patients.

To reach your destination of a LifeSmile you must first start the journey! To get your journey started visit www.lifesmiles.us/journey today!

ABOUT THE AUTHOR

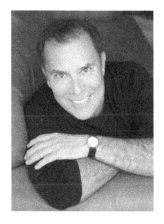

Randy Mitchmore, DDS, is the owner of LifeSmiles, a state-of-the-art full-service dental practice based in Houston, Texas. He is one of the few dentists in the country to be a Master of The Academy of General Dentistry and The American Dental Implant Association, and hold certification to give IV Sedation for any dental procedure—from dental cleaning to cosmetic work to implant surgery. A respected dental author and lecturer, he has been named one of the 'Top Dentists' by the American Registry annually since 2003.

Dr. Mitchmore completes more than *500 hours* of Continuing Education per year to stay current with cutting-edge developments in dentistry and to offer them to his patients. When he isn't busy giving them superb smiles, he is giving a smile to his community. He spent many years on the board of directors for Bering Omega Community Services, a service that provides compassionate healthcare and social services to people living with HIV/AIDS. He volunteers for Give Back a Smile, the American Academy of Cosmetic Dentistry's project to restore the broken and damaged teeth of survivors of domestic violence. In 2008, he was appointed to the Board of Trustees of the American Academy of Cosmetic Dentistry Charitable Foundation.

He has served as a Cubmaster, Rotary International President, and Paul Harris Fellow, director of a bank, Chairman of the Board of Cleveland Regional Medical Center, Chambers of Commerce, Tri-

County Mental Health and Mental Retardation, leadership roles in both United Methodist and Episcopal Churches, and is currently vice-Chair of the Montrose Management District.

Dr. Mitchmore is also the author of *10 Essential Dental Facts to Save Your Teeth*.

www.ingramcontent.com/pod-product-compliance
Lightning Source LLC
Jackson TN
JSHW011939131224
75386JS00041B/1459